MW01493986

Edited by:

Eleftherios Mylonakis, MD
Massachusetts General Hospital
Harvard University
Boston, MA

Josiah D. Rich, MD, MPH
The Miriam Hospital
Brown University
Providence, RI

Major contributor:

Brian P. Dickinson
Mount Sinai School of Medicine
New York, NY

Editorial Director: Tony Howell
Production Editor: Tony Vitale
Graphic Designer: Susan Moore-Stevenson
President/Publishing Director: Sarah Howell
VP Group Publisher: Jo Ann Kalaka-Adams
Founder: Louis Le Jacq

ISBN 1-929660-01-4

Printed in the United States of America.

Table of Contents

e. Cholecystitis/Cholangitis

f. Common Cold

g. Endocarditis

h. Erythema Migrans

n. Onychomycosis

o. Pancreatitis

p. Pelvic Inflammatory Disease

q. Peritonitis

r. Pneumonia

s. Sepsis/Immunoprophylaxis

t. Sexually Transmitted Diseases

u. Sinusitis

v. Surgical Wound Infections

w. Urethritis

x. Urinary Tract Infection

2. Pathogens
a. Aspergillosis

b. Atypical Mycobacterial Infections

c. Blastomycosis

d. Blastomycosis/Histoplasmosis

e. Brucellosis

f. Candidiasis

k. Condylomata Acuminata

l. Cryptosporidiosis

m. Cyclosporidiosis

n. Cysticercosis

o. Cytomegalovirus Infections

p. Diphtheria

q. Echinococcosis

r. Enterococcal Infections

s. Fungi

t. Gonorrhea

u. Helicobacter Pylori Infection

v. Herpes Simplex Virus Infections

w. Herpes Simplex/Herpes Zoster Virus Infections

cc. Leprosy

dd. Lyme Disease

ee. Malaria

ff. Measles

gg. Pertussis

hh. Pseudomonas Infections

ii. Respiratory Syncytial Virus Infection

jj. Rotavirus Infections

kk. Salmonellosis

ll. Schistosomiasis

mm. Shigellosis

nn. Staphylococcal Infections

oo. Streptococcal Infections

pp. Strongyloidiasis

qq. Toxoplasmosis

rr. Traveler's Diarrhea

ss. Trichomoniasis

tt. Tuberculosis

3. Infections in Special Hosts
a. Infections in Immunocompromised Patients

b. Infections in Organ Transplant Recipients

c. Infections in Patients with Diabetes

d. Infections in the Elderly

e. Neonatal Infections

f. Neutropenic Fever

4. Use of Antibiotics

5. Ongoing Trials
a. Community-Acquired Pneumonia

b. Cystitis

c. Cytomegalovirus Disease

d. Entercoccal Endocarditis

e. Enterococci

f. Enterococcus Faecium

g. Fungal Burn Wound Infections

h. Haemophilus Influnenza

i. Intra-Abdominal Infections

j. Nosocomial Infections

k. Oral or Intravenous Antibiotics

l. Otitis Media

m. Peritonitis

n. Pertussis

o. Pneumococcal Resistance

p. Pseudomonas Aeruginosa Bacteremia

q. Staphylococcus Aureus

r. Staphylococcal Infective Endocarditis

s. Urinary Tract Infections

t. Varicella

Introduction

In the past decade, major changes in the understanding of disease pathogenesis and treatment have lead to a wealth of clinical trials. *Infectious Disease Trials Review* is intended to review recent controlled clinical trials which have, or are likely to have, a significant impact on infectious disease practice. We have included only studies published in English and concentrated mainly on recent publications. This review does not include any trials on HIV or AIDS treatment. The text is divided into major headings, including specific pathogens and clinical syndromes. We have also included a section describing ongoing clinical trials.

Any review of this nature and size requires that many studies will not be included. However, this book should give a broad overview of current research activity in the field of clinical infectious diseases.

Selection of all the studies in *Infectious Disease Trials Review* reflects the totally independent judgement of the Editors. The medications, indications, and dosages for medications may or may not be approved by the Food and Drug Administration (FDA). Physicians should consult package inserts and/or a *Physician's Desk Reference* (PDR) for drug indication, contra-indications, and dosages as recommended.

We dedicate this book to our wives, Polyxeni and Pat, and children, Zoe-Stella, Nicholas and Nola for their tireless support and love. We also thank Brian P. Dickinson for his major contributions.

Thank you.

Sincerely,
Eleftherios Mylonakis, MD
Josiah D. Rich, MD, MPH

September, 2001

1. Syndromes

a. Bacteremia/Sepsis

Long-Term Survival and Function After Suspected Gram-Negative Sepsis

Title	Long-term survival and function after suspected gram-negative sepsis.
Authors	Perl TM, Dvorak L, Hwang T, et al.
Reference	JAMA 1995;274:338–345.
Disease/ Pathogen	Bacteremia/Sepsis.
Purpose	To determine the long-term (>3 months) survival of septic patients, to develop mathematical models that predict patients likely to survive long-term, and to measure the health and functional status of surviving patients.
Design	A double blind, placebo controlled efficacy trial of monoclonal antiendotoxin antibody.
Patients	A total of 103 patients with suspected gram-negative sepsis.
Follow-up	100 patients were followed for 7667 patient-months. The determinants of long-term survival (up to 6 years) were identified through two Cox proportional hazard regression models: One that included patient characteristics identified at the time of sepsis (bedside model) and another that included bedside, infection-related, and treatment characteristics (overall model).

Results

Of the 60 patients in the cohort who died at a median interval of 30.5 days after sepsis, 32 died within the first month of the septic episode, seven died within 3 months, and four more died within 6 months. In the bedside multivariate model constructed to predict long-term survival, large hazard ratios (HRs) were associated with severity of underlying illness as classified by McCabe and Jackson criteria (for rapidly fatal disease, HR=30.4, p<0.001; for ultimately fatal disease, HR=7.6, p<0.001) and the use of vasopressors (HR=2.5, p=0.001). In the overall model for long-term survival, severity of underlying illness (rapidly fatal disease HR=23.7, p<0.001; ultimately fatal disease, HR=6.5, p<0.001), number of active comorbid illnesses (HR=1.3, p=0.04), use of vasopressors at the time of sepsis (HR=2.0; p=0.02) and development of adult respiratory distress syndrome (HR=2.3; p=0.02) predicted patients most likely to die. The Acute Physiology and Chronic Health Evaluation II score was not a significant predictor of outcome when either model included the simpler McCabe and Jackson classification of underlying disease severity. We compared the health status scores with norms for the general population and found that patients with resolved sepsis reported more physical dysfunction (p<0.001), including problems with work and activities of daily living (p=0.02), and more poorly perceived general health (p<0.01). In contrast, patients' score for perceived emotional health were higher than those in the general population (p=0.004). The mean Barthel score of our patients was 85 (100=total independence) and the mean Eastern Cooperative Oncology Group score was 0.7 (0=normal, 4=100% bedridden), suggesting that the patients' physical function was not normal.

Conclusion

At the onset of suspected gram-negative sepsis, severity of underlying illness and in-hospital use of vasopressors are strong and consistent predictors of short- and long-term survival. Our data validate the McCabe and Jackson severity of illness scoring system for predicting long-term survival after sepsis. Physical dysfunction and more poorly perceived general health occur commonly after sepsis.

1. Syndromes

b. Bronchitis/Pneumonia

***Decreasing Antibiotic Use in Ambulatory Practice:
Impact of a Multidimensional Intervention on the Treatment
of Uncomplicated Acute Bronchitis in Adults.***

Title	Decreasing antibiotic use in ambulatory practice: Impact of a multidimensional intervention on the treatment of uncomplicated acute bronchitis in adults.
Authors	Gonzales R, Steiner JF, Lum A, et al.
Reference	JAMA 1999;281:1512–1519.
Disease/ Pathogen	Bronchitis.
Purpose	To decrease total antibiotic use for uncomplicated acute bronchitis in adults.
Design	Prospective, nonrandomized controlled trial, including baseline (November 1996–February 1997) and study (November 1997–February 1998) periods.
Patients	Consecutive adults diagnosed as having uncomplicated acute bronchitis. A total of 2462 adults were included at baseline and 2027 adults were included in the study. Clinicians included 56 physicians, 28 physician assistants or nurse practitioners, and 9 registered nurses.
Follow-up	Antibiotic prescriptions for uncomplicated acute bronchitis during baseline and study periods.
Treatment/ prophylaxis regimen	The full intervention site received household and office-based patient educational materials, as well as a clinician intervention consisting of education, practice-profiling, and academic detailing. A limited intervention site received only office-based educational materials, and control sites provided usual care.

Decreasing Antibiotic Use in Ambulatory Practice: Impact of a Multidimensional Intervention on the Treatment of Uncomplicated Acute Bronchitis in Adults.

(continued)

Results	Antibiotic prescription rates for uncomplicated acute bronchitis were similar at all four sites during the baseline period. During the study period, there was a substantial decline in antibiotic prescription rates at the full intervention site (from 74% to 48%, p=0.003), but not at the control and limited intervention sites (78% to 76%, p=0.81, and 82% to 77%, p=0.68, respectively). Compared with control sites, changes in nonantibiotic prescriptions (inhaled bronchodilators, cough suppressants, and analgesics) were not significantly different for intervention sites. Return office visits (within 30 days of the incident visit) for bronchitis or pneumonia did not change significantly for any of the sites.
Conclusion	Antibiotic treatment of adults diagnosed as having uncomplicated acute bronchitis can be safely reduced using a combination of patient and clinician interventions.

Efficacy of Oral Ciprofloxacin Vs Clarithromycin for Treatment of Acute Bacterial Exacerbations of Chronic Bronchitis. The Bronchitis Study Group

Title	Efficacy of oral ciprofloxacin vs clarithromycin for treatment of acute bacterial exacerbations of chronic bronchitis. The Bronchitis Study Group.
Authors	Chodosh S, Schreurs A, Siami G, et al.
Reference	Clin Infect Dis 1998;27(4):730–738.
Disease/ Pathogen	Bronchitis.
Purpose	To compare the efficacy of ciprofloxacin with that of clarithromycin as therapy for patients with acute bacterial exacerbations of chronic bronchitis (ABECB) from whom a pretherapy pathogen was isolated.
Design	Prospective, multicenter, double blind study.
Patients	Three hundred seventy-six patients with acute exacerbations of chronic bronchitis were enrolled in the study; 234 had an ABECB.
Follow-up	The efficacy was measured by the infection-free interval. Clinical and microbiological responses at the end of therapy were secondary efficacy variables.
Treatment/ prophylaxis regimen	Patients randomly received either ciprofloxacin or clarithromycin (500 mg twice a day for 14 days).

Efficacy of Oral Ciprofloxacin Vs Clarithromycin for Treatment of Acute Bacterial Exacerbations of Chronic Bronchitis. The Bronchitis Study Group

(continued)

Results	Clinical resolution was observed in 90% of ciprofloxacin recipients and 82% of clarithromycin recipients for whom efficacy could be evaluated. The median infection-free interval was 142 days for ciprofloxacin recipients and 51 days for clarithromycin recipients ($p=0.15$). Bacteriologic eradication rates were 91% for ciprofloxacin recipients and 77% for clarithromycin recipients ($p=0.01$).
Conclusion	Compared with clarithromycin, treatment of ABECB with ciprofloxacin was associated with a trend toward a longer infection-free interval and a statistically significantly higher bacteriologic eradication rate.

Randomized, Double Blind Study of Ciprofloxacin and Cefuroxime Axetil for Treatment of Acute Bacterial Exacerbations of Chronic Bronchitis

Title	Randomized, double blind study of ciprofloxacin and cefuroxime axetil for treatment of acute bacterial exacerbations of chronic bronchitis.
Authors	Chodosh S, McCarty J, Farkas S, et al.
Reference	Clin Infect Dis 1998;27(4):722-729.
Disease/ Pathogen	Bronchitis.
Purpose	To compare the interval to clinical relapse in patients with acute bacterial exacerbations of chronic bronchitis following treatment with ciprofloxacin or cefuroxime axetil.
Design	Prospective, double blind, multicenter.
Patients	Three hundred seven patients with acute exacerbations of chronic bronchitis were enrolled; 208 had an exacerbation due to a bacterial pathogen.
Follow-up	Clinical and microbiological responses at the end of therapy were secondary efficacy.
Treatment/ prophylaxis regimen	Outpatients randomly received either ciprofloxacin or cefuroxime axetil (500 mg twice a day for 14 days).

(continued)

Results	Clinical resolution at the end of ciprofloxacin and cefuroxime axetil therapy for patients for whom efficacy could be evaluated was 93% and 90%, respectively. Bacteriologic eradication rates were statistically higher for ciprofloxacin recipients (96% [89 of 93]) than for cefuroxime axetil recipients (82% [80 of 97]) (p<0.01). The median infection-free interval was 146 days for ciprofloxacin recipients vs 178 days for cefuroxime axetil recipients (p=0.37).
Conclusion	Ciprofloxacin was associated with an infection-free interval and clinical response that were similar to those associated with cefuroxime axetil, but the bacteriologic eradication rate associated with ciprofloxacin was statistically significantly higher than that associated with cefuroxime axetil.

Dosing of Amoxicillin/Clavulanate Given Every 12 Hours Is as Effective as Dosing Every 8 Hours for Treatment of Lower Respiratory Tract Infection

Title	Dosing of amoxicillin/clavulanate given every 12 hours is as effective as dosing every 8 hours for treatment of lower respiratory tract infection.
Authors	Calver AD, Walsh NS, Quinn PF, et al.
Reference	Clin Infect Dis 1997;24(4):570–574.
Disease/ Pathogen	Lower respiratory tract infections.
Purpose	To compare the efficacy of amoxicillin/clavulanate given every 12 hours to every 8 hours for the treatment of lower respiratory tract infections.
Design	In this double blind study, 557 patients with lower respiratory tract infection were randomly assigned to receive amoxicillin/clavulanate orally either every 8 or 12 hours.
Patients	557 patients with lower respiratory tract infection.
Follow-up	7–15 days.
Treatment/ prophylaxis regimen	Patients were randomly assigned to receive amoxicillin/clavulanate orally either every 12 hours (875/125 mg) or every 8 hours (500/125 mg) for 7–15 days.

Dosing of Amoxicillin/Clavulanate Given Every 12 Hours Is as Effective as Dosing Every 8 Hours for Treatment of Lower Respiratory Tract Infection

(continued)

Results

For the 455 patients evaluable for clinical efficacy at the end of therapy, clinical success was similar in the two groups: 93% and 94% in the 12-hour and 8-hour groups, respectively (p=0.42). Bacteriologic success at the end of therapy was also comparable: 97% and 91% in the 12-hour and 8-hour groups, respectively (p=0.86). The occurrence of adverse events related to treatment was similar for the two groups, but fewer patients in the 12-hour group reported moderate or severe diarrhea.

Conclusion

Amoxicillin/clavulanate (875/125 mg) given every 12 hours is as effective and safe as every 8-hour-administration of the combination (500/125 mg) for the treatment of lower respiratory tract infection.

1. Syndromes

c. Catheter-Related Infections

A Comparison of Two Antimicrobial-Impregnated Central Venous Catheters

Title	A comparison of two antimicrobial-impregnated central venous catheters.
Authors	Darouiche RO, Raad II, Heard SO, et al.
Reference	N Engl J Med 1999;340:1-8.
Disease/ Pathogen	Catheter colonization and systemic infections.
Purpose	To compare catheters impregnated with minocycline and rifampin with those impregnated with chlorhexidine and silver sulfadiazine, in terms of the rates of colonization of catheters and bloodstream infection.
Design	Prospective, randomized, clinical trial, multicenter.
Patients	865 study catheters (414 impregnated with minocycline and rifampin, and 451 impregnated with chlorhexidine and silver sulfadiazine) were inserted into 817 patients who were at high risk for catheter-related infection (such as patients in intensive care units or those who were immunocompromised) and were likely to require a central venous catheter for three or more days were eligible for the study.
Treatment/ prophylaxis regimen	Insertion of polyurethane, triple-lumen catheters impregnated with either minocycline and rifampin (on both the luminal and external surfaces) or chlorhexidine and silver sulfadiazine (on only the external surface).

Results

Of 865 catheters inserted, 738 (85 %) produced culture results that could be evaluated. The clinical characteristics of the patients and the risk factors for infection were similar in the two groups. Catheters impregnated with minocycline and rifampin were one third as likely to be colonized as catheters impregnated with chlorhexidine and silver sulfadiazine (28 of 356 catheters [7.9%] vs 87 of 382 [22.8%], p<0.001), and catheter-related bloodstream infection was one twelfth as likely in catheters impregnated with minocycline and rifampin (1 of 356 [0.3%], vs 13 of 382 [3.4%] for those impregnated with chlorhexidine and silver sulfadiazine; p<0.002).

Conclusion

The use of central venous catheters impregnated with minocycline and rifampin is associated with a lower rate of infection than the use of catheters impregnated with chlorhexidine and silver sulfadiazine.

Prevention of Central Venous Catheter-Related Bloodstream Infection by Use of an Antiseptic-Impregnated Catheter: A Randomized, Controlled Trial.

Title	Prevention of central venous catheter-related bloodstream infection by use of an antiseptic-impregnated catheter: A randomized, controlled trial.
Authors	Maki DG, Stolz SM, Wheeler S, et al.
Reference	Ann Intern Med 1997;127:257–266.
Disease/ Pathogen	Catheter colonization and systemic infections.
Purpose	To determine 1) the efficacy of a novel antiseptic catheter in preventing central venous catheter-related infection, 2) patient tolerance of this catheter, and 3) the sources of bloodstream infection originating from noncuffed, multi-lumen central venous catheters.
Design	Randomized, controlled clinical trial.
Patients	158 adults scheduled to receive a central venous catheter; 403 catheters were studied.
Treatment/ prophylaxis regimen	Participants received either a standard triple-lumen polyurethane catheter or a catheter that was indistinguishable from the standard catheter and was impregnated with chlorhexidine and silver sulfadiazine.

Prevention of Central Venous Catheter-Related Bloodstream Infection by Use of an Antiseptic-Impregnated Catheter: A Randomized, Controlled Trial.

(continued)

Results

Antiseptic catheters were less likely to be colonized at removal than control catheters (13.5 compared with 24.1 colonized catheters per 100 catheters; relative risk, 0.56 [95% CI 0.36–0.89]; p=0.005) and were nearly fivefold less likely to produce bloodstream infection (1.0 compared with 4.7 infections per 100 catheters; 1.6 compared with 7.6 infections per 1000 catheter-days; relative risk, 0.21 [CI 0.03–0.95]; p=0.03). In the control group, 8 catheter-related bloodstream infections were caused by staphylococcus aureus, gram-negative bacilli, enterococci, or Candida species; no infections with these organisms occurred in the antiseptic catheter group (p=0.003). No adverse effects from the antiseptic catheter were seen, and none of the 122 isolates obtained from infected catheters in either group showed in vitro resistance to chlorhexidine-silver sulfadiazine. Cost-benefit analysis indicated that the antiseptic catheter should prove cost-beneficial if an institution's rate of catheter-related bacteremia with noncuffed central venous catheters is at least three infections per 1000 catheter days.

Conclusion

The chlorhexidine-silver sulfadiazine catheter is well tolerated, reduces the incidence of catheter-related infection, extends the time that noncuffed central venous catheters can be safely left in place for the short term, and should allow cost savings.

The Pathogenesis and Epidemiology of Catheter-Related Infection with Pulmonary Artery Swan-Ganz Catheters: A Prospective Study Utilizing Molecular Subtyping.

Title	The pathogenesis and epidemiology of catheter-related infection with pulmonary artery Swan-Ganz catheters: A prospective study utilizing molecular subtyping.
Authors	Mermel LA, McCormick RD, Springman SR, et al.
Reference	Am J Med 1991;91(3B):197S–205S.
Disease/ Pathogen	Catheter-related infection.
Purpose	To delineate the pathogenesis and epidemiology of catheter-related infection with Swan-Ganz pulmonary artery (PA) catheters.
Design	A prospective clinical study of hospitalized adult medical and surgical patients was done.
Follow-up	Role of catheter material was assessed by randomizing insertions to heparin-bonded PA catheters made of polyvinylchloride or polyurethane. Sources of infection and pathogenesis were studied by culturing skin, the introducer, the PA catheter tip, all hubs, infusate from each lumen, and the extravascular portion of the PA catheter beneath the external protective plastic sleeve. Concordance between isolates from sources and infected catheters was determined by speciation, antibiogram, and for coagulase-negative staphylococci, plasmid profile analysis.

The Pathogenesis and Epidemiology of Catheter-Related Infection with Pulmonary Artery Swan-Ganz Catheters: A Prospective Study Utilizing Molecular Subtyping.

(continued)

Results

Overall, 65 (22%) of 297 Swan-Ganz catheters showed local infection of the introducer (58 catheters) or the intravascular portion of the PA catheter (20 catheters); only two catheters (0.7%) caused bacteremia. Eighty percent of infected Swan-Ganz catheters (the introducer or PA catheter) showed concordance with organisms cultured from skin of the insertion site, 17% with a contaminated hub and 18% with organisms contaminating the extravascular portion of the PA catheter beneath the sleeve. Isolates from infected PA catheters were most likely to show concordance with concomitantly infected introducers (71%). Cutaneous colonization of the insertion site with greater than 10^2 cfu/10 cm^2 (relative risk [RR] 5.5; p<0.001), insertion into an internal jugular vein (RR 4.3; p<0.01), catheterization >3 days (RR 3.1; p<0.01), and insertion in the operating room using less stringent barrier precautions (RR 2.1; p=0.03) were each associated with a significantly increased risk of catheter-related infection. The risk of bacteremic infection with Swan-Ganz catheters is now low, in the range of 1%, with reasonable care. Swan-Ganz catheters are vulnerable to contamination from multiple sources, but the patient's skin is the single most important source of organisms causing invasive infection, which in most cases, involves the introducer rather than the PA catheter. Heavy colonization of the insertion site, percutaneous insertion in the internal jugular vein rather than subclavian vein, catheterization longer than 3 days, and insertion with less stringent barrier precautions significantly increase the risk of catheter-related infection.

Conclusion

These findings hold promise for application to management of Swan-Ganz catheters and research in catheter design to reduce the risk of catheter-related infection.

1. Syndromes

d. Cervicitis/Urethritis

Minocycline Compared with Doxycycline in the Treatment of Nongonococcal Urethritis and Mucopurulent Cervicitis

Title	Minocycline compared with doxycycline in the treatment of nongonococcal urethritis and mucopurulent cervicitis.
Authors	Romanowski B, Talbot H, Stadnyk M, et al.
Reference	Ann Intern Med 1993;119:16–22.
Disease/ Pathogen	Nongonococcal urethritis and cervicitis.
Purpose	To compare the efficacy and tolerability of minocycline vs doxycycline in the treatment of nongonococcal urethritis and mucopurulent cervicitis.
Design	Randomized, double blind trial.
Patients	151 men and 102 women with nongonococcal urethritis, mucopurulent cervicitis or whose sexual partner had either condition, or a positive culture for Chlamydia trachomatis.
Follow-up	7 weeks.
Treatment/ prophylaxis regimen	Minocycline, 100 mg nightly, or doxycycline, 100 mg twice daily, each administered for 7 days.

(continued)

Results

253 patients were enrolled (133 doxycycline; 120 minocycline). Chlamydia trachomatis was initially isolated from 31% of men and 39% of women. Men with a positive smear had a higher symptom/sign score ($p<0.001$) and were more likely to have chlamydia ($p=0.004$). Positive endocervical smears were not associated with symptoms or signs ($p>0.2$) but correlated with isolation of chlamydia ($p<0.001$). One hundred sixty-two patients (64%) completed the study. The proportion with urethritis or cervicitis did not differ by treatment group at any follow-up visit ($p>0.08$). Unprotected sexual contact did not affect clinical or microbiological cure rates. Adverse effects occurred more frequently in the doxycycline group (men: 43% vs 26%; $p=0.05$; women: 62% vs 35%; $p=0.009$). Although the proportion with dizziness did not differ by drug administered ($p=0.1$), dizziness was reported more often by women (11% vs 3%).

Conclusion

Minocycline, 100 mg nightly, was as effective as doxycycline, 100 mg twice daily, each given for 7 days in the treatment of nongonococcal urethritis and mucopurulent cervicitis. Vomiting and gastrointestinal upset occurred more frequently in the doxycycline group.

1. Syndromes

e. Cholecystitis/Cholangitis

Piperacillin to Prevent Cholangitis after Endoscopic Retrograde Cholangiopancreatography: A Randomized, Controlled Trial.

Title	Piperacillin to prevent cholangitis after endoscopic retrograde cholangiopancreatography: A randomized, controlled trial.
Authors	van den Hazel SJ, Speelman P, Dankert J, et al.
Reference	Ann Intern Med 1996;125:442–447.
Disease/Pathogen	Cholangitis.
Purpose	To determine the efficacy of single-dose antibiotic prophylaxis with piperacillin for Endoxopic Retrograde Cholangiopancreatography- (ERCP) induced cholangitis.
Design	Randomized, double blind, placebo controlled, clinical trial.
Patients	Patients who had ERCP for suspected biliary tract stones or distal common bile duct stricture were eligible.
Follow-up	1 week.
Treatment/prophylaxis regimen	Piperacillin, 4 g, or placebo was given intravenously approximately 30 minutes before ERCP.

*Piperacillin to Prevent Cholangitis after Endoscopic
Retrograde Cholangiopancreatography:
A Randomized, Controlled Trial.*

(continued)

Results   551 consecutive patients were enrolled. During ERCP,
           stones were found in 147 patients, malignant distal stric-
           tures were found in 203 patients, other pathologic find-
           ings were seen in 88 patients, and normal biliary tracts
           were seen in 113 patients. 17 of the 281 patients who
           received placebo (6%) and 12 of the 270 patients who
           received piperacillin (4.4%) developed acute cholangitis
           (relative risk, 0.73 [95% confidence interval [CI] 0.36 to
           1.51]). The absolute risk reduction was 1.6% (CI -5.3% to
           2.1%). All cases of cholangitis (with the exception of one
           case seen in a patient in the piperacillin group) were mild
           or moderate in severity.

Conclusion Single-dose prophylaxis with piperacillin is not associated
           with a clinically significant reduction in the incidence of
           acute cholangitis after ERCP in patients suspected of hav-
           ing biliary tract stones or distal common bile duct stricture.

1. Syndromes

f. Common Cold

Effectiveness and Safety of Intranasal Ipratropium Bromide in Common Colds: A Randomized, Double Blind, Placebo Controlled Trial.

Title	Effectiveness and safety of intranasal ipratropium bromide in common colds: A randomized, double blind, placebo controlled trial.
Authors	Hayden FG, Diamond L, Wood PB, et al.
Reference	Ann Intern Med 1996;125:89–97.
Disease/ Pathogen	Common cold.
Purpose	To determine the tolerability and clinical effectiveness of intranasal ipratropium bromide for the treatment of symptoms of common colds.
Design	Randomized, double blind, placebo controlled trial, multicenter.
Patients	411 previously healthy persons 14 to 56 years of age who had cold symptoms that lasted for no more than 36 hours, rhinorrhea subjectively judged to be of at least moderate severity, and documented nasal discharge of at least 1.5 g over a 1-hour observation period.
Follow-up	5 days.

Effectiveness and Safety of Intranasal Ipratropium Bromide in Common Colds: A Randomized, Double Blind, Placebo Controlled Trial

(continued)

Treatment/ prophylaxis regimen	Either 1) ipratropium bromide nasal spray 0.06% in buffered salt solution, two 42-microgram sprays per nostril administered by metered pump spray; 2) control nasal spray, which consisted of buffered salt solution; or 3) no treatment. Treatments were self-administered three or four times daily during waking hours for 4 days. After receiving their morning dose, patients stayed at the study center for 6 hours on study day 1, and 3 hours on study day 2; symptom severity was recorded and nasal mucus discharges were collected and weighed hourly during these periods.
Results	Ipratropium recipients had 26% less nasal discharge than controls (p=0.0024), and 34% less nasal discharge than untreated patients (p=0.0001). Severity of rhinorrhea as judged subjectively was reduced in ipratropium recipients by 31% compared with controls, and by 78% compared with untreated patients (p=0.0001 for both comparisons). In addition to being associated with reductions in daily assessments of the severity of rhinorrhea (p≤0.003), ipratropium was associated with reduced sneezing on study days 2 (20% difference; p=0.03) and 4 (30% difference; p=0.02) but not with reduced nasal congestion compared with the control spray. Ipratropium was generally well tolerated but was associated with higher rates of blood-tinged mucous (16.8% in the ipratropium group, compared with 3.6% in the control group; p=0.01) and nasal dryness (11.7% in the ipratropium group compared with 3.6% in the control group; p=0.021) than the control spray. Patient assessments of the overall effectiveness of treatment were more favorable for ipratropium than for the control spray (p≤0.026) or for no treatment (p≤0.002) on each day of inquiry (study days 1, 2, and 5).
Conclusion	Intranasal ipratropium bromide provides specific relief of rhinorrhea and sneezing associated with common colds.

Zinc Gluconate Lozenges for Treating the Common Cold: A Randomized, Double Blind, Placebo Controlled Study.

Title	Zinc gluconate lozenges for treating the common cold: A randomized, double blind, placebo controlled study.
Authors	Mossad SB, Macknin ML, Mendendorp SV, et al.
Reference	Ann Intern Med 1996;125:81–88.
Disease/ Pathogen	Common Cold.
Purpose	To test the efficacy of zinc gluconate lozenges in reducing the duration of symptoms caused by the common cold.
Design	Randomized, double blind, placebo controlled study.
Patients	100 employees of the Cleveland Clinic who developed symptoms of the common cold within 24 hours before enrollment.
Follow-up	18 days.
Treatment/ prophylaxis regimen	Patients in the zinc group (n=50) received lozenges (one lozenge every 2 hours while awake) containing 13.3 mg of zinc from zinc gluconate as long as they had cold symptoms. Patients in the placebo group (n=50) received similarly administered lozenges that contained 5% calcium lactate pentahydrate instead of zinc gluconate.

Results   The time to complete resolution of symptoms was signif-
              icantly shorter in the zinc group than in the placebo
              group (median, 4.4 days compared with 7.6 days;
              p<0.001). The zinc group had significantly fewer days
              with coughing (median, 2 days compared with 4.5 days;
              p=0.04), headache (2 days and 3 days; p=0.02), hoarse-
              ness (2 days and 3 days; p=0.02), nasal congestion (4 days
              and 6 days; p=0.002), nasal drainage (4 days and 7 days;
              p<0.001), and sore throat (1 day and 3 days; p<0.001). The
              groups did not differ significantly in the resolution of
              fever, muscle ache, scratchy throat, or sneezing. More
              patients in the zinc group than in the placebo group had
              side effects (90% compared with 62%; p<0.001), nausea
              (20% compared with 4%; p=0.02), and bad-taste reactions
              (80% compared with 30%; p<0.001).

Conclusion   Zinc gluconate in the form and dosage studied signifi-
              cantly reduced the duration of symptoms of the common
              cold. The mechanism of action of this substance in treat-
              ing the common cold remains unknown. Individual
              patients must decide whether the possible beneficial
              effects of zinc gluconate on cold symptoms outweigh the
              possible adverse effects.

1. Syndromes

g. Endocarditis

Treatment of Streptococcal Endocarditis with a Single Daily Dose of Ceftriaxone Sodium for 4 Weeks. Efficacy and Outpatient Treatment Feasibility

Title	Treatment of streptococcal endocarditis with a single daily dose of ceftriaxone sodium for 4 weeks. Efficacy and outpatient treatment feasibility.
Authors	Francioli P, Etienne J, Hoigne R, et al.
Reference	JAMA 1992;267:264–267.
Disease/ Pathogen	Endocarditis.
Purpose	To evaluate the efficacy and safety of ceftriaxone sodium in the treatment of streptococcal endocarditis.
Design	An open, multicenter, noncomparative study with a follow-up of patients for 4 months to 5 years.
Patients	59 patients with defined criteria for streptococcal endocarditis.
Follow-up	Clinical outcome and microbiological cure rate.
Treatment/ prophylaxis regimen	Ceftriaxone sodium administered at a once-daily dose of 2 g for 4 weeks.

(continued)

Results	Among the 59 patients, 55 completed the treatment and were followed up for 4 months to 5 years. No patients showed evidence of relapse. Treatment was completely uneventful in 42 patients (71%). A cardiac valve was replaced in four patients (7%) receiving antimicrobial therapy and in six patients (10%) who had completed antimicrobial therapy. One of the 10 valves taken for culture at surgery was positive, but only for micro-organisms that were different from the micro-organism isolated before the treatment. The treatment had to be interrupted in four patients because of drug allergy. Other side effects were mild, except for two cases of reversible neutropenia. The treatment was easy to administer: 27 patients (46%) had no permanent intravenous catheter at any time, seven patients (12%) had such a catheter for less than 4 days. 23 patients (39%) were discharged from the hospital less than 2 weeks after admission.
Conclusion	Ceftriaxone sodium administered at a once-daily dose of 2 g appears to be an effective and safe treatment of streptococcal endocarditis. In hospitals, this agent may be more convenient to administer than penicillin G with or without aminoglycosides. Some patients may even be treated as outpatients.

Treatment of Streptococcal Endocarditis with a Single Daily Dose of Ceftriaxone and Netilmicin for 14 Days: A Prospective, Multicenter Study.

Title	Treatment of streptococcal endocarditis with a single daily dose of ceftriaxone and netilmicin for 14 days: A prospective, multicenter study.
Authors	Francioli P, Ruch W, Stamboulian D.
Reference	Clin Infect Dis 1995;21(6):1406–1410.
Disease/ Pathogen	Endocarditis.
Purpose	To evaluate a 2 week-course of ceftriaxone plus netilmicin for the treatment of streptococcal endocarditis.
Design	Multicenter, prospective, open label.
Patients	Of the 52 patients with endocarditis, 31 were infected with viridans streptococci, 18 with Streptococcus bovis, two with Gemella morbillorum, and one with group C streptococcus; 48 patients were assessable.
Treatment/ prophylaxis regimen	A 2-week course of ceftriaxone (2 g) plus netilmicin (4 mg/kg) was administered as one short daily IV infusion.

Treatment of Streptococcal Endocarditis with a Single Daily Dose of Ceftriaxone and Netilmicin for 14 Days: A Prospective, Multicenter Study.

(continued)

Results   Infection was cured in 42 cases, 35 treated medically and seven treated both medically and surgically. Five patients died without evidence of active infection, and one relapsed. The bacteriologic failure was due to a strain of G. morbillorum against which no synergy of ceftriaxone and netilmicin was evident in vitro. The serum creatinine level increased during treatment in four cases, all involving patients >65 years old who had renal risk factors; in two of these cases, values did not return to baseline during follow-up. Of 40 patients assessed for auditory function, only one developed decreased perception of borderline significance. Other adverse reactions were mild.

Conclusion   The authors conclude that this regimen was efficacious, safe, and cost-effective for the treatment of streptococcal endocarditis. However, it must be used with caution for patients with pre-existing renal impairment or concomitant exposure to other potentially nephrotoxic agents.

Oral Antibiotic Treatment of Right-Sided Staphylococcal Endocarditis in Injection Drug Users: Prospective, Randomized Comparison with Parenteral Therapy.

Title	Oral antibiotic treatment of right-sided staphylococcal endocarditis in injection drug users: Prospective randomized comparison with parenteral therapy.
Authors	Heldman AW, Hartert TV, Ray SC, et al.
Reference	Am J Med 1996;101(1):68–76.
Disease/ Pathogen	Right-sided staphylococcal endocarditis.
Purpose	To compare the efficacy and safety of inpatient oral antibiotic treatment (oral) vs standard parenteral antibiotic treatment (intravenous) for right-sided staphylococcal endocarditis in injection drug users.
Design	Prospective, randomized, nonblinded trial.
Patients	Febrile injection drug users.
Follow-up	Test-of-cure blood cultures were obtained during inpatient observation 6 and 7 days after the completion of antibiotic therapy, and again at outpatient follow-up 1 month later.
Treatment/ prophylaxis regimen	Patients were assigned to begin oral or intravenous (IV) treatment on admission, before blood culture results were available. Oral therapy consisted of ciprofloxacin and rifampin. Parenteral therapy was oxacillin or vancomycin, plus gentamicin for the first 5 days. Antibiotic dosing was adjusted for renal dysfunction. Bacteremic subjects having right-sided staphylococcal endocarditis received 28 days of inpatient therapy with the assigned antibiotics.

Oral Antibiotic Treatment of Right-Sided Staphylococcal Endocarditis in Injection Drug Users: Prospective, Randomized Comparison with Parenteral Therapy.

(continued)

Results	Of 573 injection drug users who were hospitalized because of a febrile illness and suspected right-sided staphylococcal endocarditis, 93 subjects (16.2%) had two or more sets of blood cultures positive for staphylococci; 85 of these bacteremic subjects (14.8%) satisfied diagnostic criteria for at least possible right-sided staphylococcal endocarditis (no other source of bacteremia was apparent) and entered the trial. Forty-four (oral 19; IV, 25) of these 85 subjects completed inpatient treatment and evaluation including test-of-cure blood cultures. There were four treatment failures (oral 1 [5.2%]; IV 3 [12%]; not significant, Fisher's exact test). Drug toxicity was significantly more common in the parenterally treated group (oral 3%; IV 62%; p<0.0001), consisting largely of oxacillin-associated increases in liver enzymes.
Conclusion	For selected patients with right-sided staphylococcal endocarditis, oral ciprofloxacin plus rifampin is effective and is associated with less drug toxicity than is intravenous therapy.

Ceftriaxone Once Daily for 4 Weeks Compared with Ceftriaxone Plus Gentamicin Once Daily for 2 Weeks for Treatment of Endocarditis Due to Penicillin-Susceptible Streptococci

Title	Ceftriaxone once daily for 4 weeks compared with ceftriaxone plus gentamicin once daily for 2 weeks for treatment of endocarditis due to penicillin-susceptible streptococci.
Authors	Sexton DJ, Tenenbaum MJ, Wilson WR, et al.
Reference	Clin Infect Dis 1998;27(6):1470–1474.
Disease/ Pathogen	Endocarditis.
Purpose	To compare the efficacy and safety of ceftriaxone with the combination therapy ceftriaxone and gentamicin for endocarditis due to penicillin-susceptible streptococci.
Design	Randomized, multicenter, open label study. 61 patients were enrolled in the study.
Patients	51 evaluable patients with endocarditis.
Follow-up	3 months.
Treatment/ prophylaxis regimen	Patients received either monotherapy with 2 g of intravenous ceftriaxone once daily for 4 weeks or combination therapy with 2 g of intravenous ceftriaxone and 3 mg of intravenous gentamicin/kg once daily for 2 weeks.

Ceftriaxone Once Daily for 4 Weeks Compared with Ceftriaxone Plus Gentamicin Once Daily for 2 Weeks for Treatment of Endocarditis Due to Penicillin-Susceptible Streptococci

(continued)

Results
Clinical cure was observed for 51 evaluable patients both at termination of therapy, and at the 3-month follow-up of 25 (96.2%) of 26 monotherapy recipients and 24 (96%) of 25 combination therapy recipients. Of the 23 patients in each treatment group who were microbiologically evaluable, 22 (95.7%) in each group were considered cured. No patient had evidence of relapse. Fourteen patients (27.5%) required cardiac surgery after initiation of treatment, including five monotherapy recipients and nine combination therapy recipients. Adverse effects were minimal in both treatment groups.

Conclusion
2 g of ceftriaxone once daily for 4 weeks and 2 g of ceftriaxone in combination with 3 mg of gentamicin/kg once daily for 2 weeks are both effective and safe for the treatment of streptococcal endocarditis.

Effectiveness of Cloxacillin with and without Gentamicin in Short-Term Therapy for Right-Sided Staphylococcus Aureus Endocarditis: A Randomized, Controlled Trial.

Title	Effectiveness of cloxacillin with and without gentamicin in short-term therapy for right-sided staphylococcus aureus endocarditis: A randomized, controlled trial.
Authors	Ribera E, Gomez-Jimenez J, Cortes E, et al.
Reference	Ann Intern Med 1996;125:969–974.
Disease/ Pathogen	Bacterial endocarditis.
Purpose	To compare the efficacy of cloxacillin alone with that of cloxacillin plus gentamicin for the 2-week treatment of right-sided S. aureus endocarditis in intravenous drug users.
Design	Open, randomized, controlled trial.
Patients	90 consecutive intravenous drug users who had isolated tricuspid valve endocarditis caused by methicillin-susceptible S. aureus.
Follow-up	6 months
Treatment/ prophylaxis regimen	Cloxacillin (2 g intravenously every 4 hours for 14 days) alone or combined with gentamicin (1 mg/kg of body weight intravenously every 8 hours for 7 days).

Effectiveness of Cloxacillin with and without Gentamicin in Short-Term Therapy for Right-Sided Staphylococcus Aureus Endocarditis: A Randomized, Controlled Trial

(continued)

Results

In an analysis of the efficacy subset, treatment was successful in 34 of the 38 patients who received cloxacillin alone (89% [95% CI 75%-97%]) and 31 of the 36 patients who received cloxacillin plus gentamicin (86% [CI 71%-95%]). Three patients died: One in the cloxacillin group and two in the combination therapy group. Of the 37 patients who completed 2-week treatment with cloxacillin, 34 (92%) were cured, and 3 (8%) needed prolonged treatment to cure the infection. Of the 34 patients who completed 2-week treatment with cloxacillin plus gentamicin, 32 (94%) were cured and 2 (6%) required treatment for 4 weeks. One patient in the combination group had relapse.

Conclusion

A penicillinase-resistant penicillin used as single-agent therapy for 2 weeks was effective for most patients with isolated tricuspid endocarditis caused by methicillin-susceptible S. aureus. Adding gentamicin did not appear to provide any therapeutic advantages. Additional studies to confirm the therapeutic equivalence of short-course therapy with penicillinase-resistant penicillin alone and therapy with combined regimens are warranted.

Prosthetic Valve Endocarditis Resulting from Nosocomial Bacteremia: A Prospective, Multicenter Study.

Title	Prosthetic valve endocarditis resulting from nosocomial bacteremia: A prospective, multicenter study.
Authors	Fang G, Keys TF, Gentry LO, et al.
Reference	Ann Intern Med 1993;119:560–567.
Disease/ Pathogen	Endocarditis.
Purpose	To determine the incidence of endocarditis in bacteremic patients with prosthetic heart valves and the risk factors for and the effect of duration of antibiotic therapy on development of endocarditis in such patients.
Design	Multicenter, prospective observational study.
Patients	171 consecutive patients with prosthetic heart valves who developed bacteremia during hospitalization.
Follow-up	12 months.

Results

Patients were evaluated when they were identified as having bacteremia and 1, 2, 6, and 12 months after its occurrence. Of 171 patients, 74 (43%) developed endocarditis: 56 (33%) had prosthetic valve endocarditis at the time bacteremia was discovered ("endocarditis at outset"), whereas 18 (11%) developed endocarditis a mean of 45 days after bacteremia was discovered ("new endocarditis"). Mitral valve location and staphylococcal bacteremia (Staphylococcus aureus or Staphylococcus epidermidis) were significantly associated with the development of "new" endocarditis. All 18 cases of new endocarditis were nosocomial, and in six of these cases (33%), bacteremia was acquired via intravascular devices. 21 patients without evidence of endocarditis at the time of bacteremia received short-term antibiotic therapy (<14 days); one patient (5%) developed endocarditis. Eleven of 70 patients (16%) who received long-term antibiotic therapy (>14 days) developed endocarditis (p>0.2).

Conclusion

Bacteremic patients with prosthetic heart valves were at notable risk for developing endocarditis, even when they received antibiotic therapy before endocarditis developed, and regardless of the duration of such therapy. Intravascular devices were a common portal of entry.

New Criteria for Diagnosis of Infective Endocarditis: Utilization of Specific Echocardiographic Findings.

Title	New criteria for diagnosis of infective endocarditis: Utilization of specific echocardiographic findings.
Authors	Durack DT, Lukes AS, Bright DK.
Reference	Am J Med 1994;96(3):200–209.
Disease/ Pathogen	Infective endocarditis.
Purpose	This study was designed to develop improved criteria for the diagnosis of infective endocarditis and compare these criteria with currently accepted criteria in a large series of cases.
Design	A total of 405 consecutive cases of suspected infective endocarditis in 353 patients evaluted in a tertiary care hospital from 1985–1992 were analyzed using new diagnostic criteria for endocarditis.
Patients	353 patients with infective endocarditis.
Follow-up	The authors defined two "major criteria" (typical blood culture and positive echocardiogram) and six "minor criteria" (predispostion, fever, vascular phenomena, immunologic phenomena, suggestive echocardiogram, and suggestive microbiologic findings). The authors defined three diagnostic categories: (1) "definite" by pathologic or clinical criteria, (2) "possible," and (3) "rejected." Each suspected case of endocarditis was classified using bothe old and new criteria. Sixty-nine pathologically proven cases were reclassified after exclusion of the surgical or autopsy findings, enabling comparison of clinical diagnostic criteria in proven cases.

Results

55 (80%) of the 69 pathologically confirmed cases were classified as clinically definite endocarditis. The older criteria classified only 35 (51%) of the 69 pathologically confirmed cases into the analogous probable category (p<0.0001). 12 (17%) pathologically confirmed cases were rejected by older clinical criteria, but none were rejected by the new criteria. 71 (21%) of the remaining 336 cases that were not proven pathologically were probable by older criteria, whereas the new criteria almost doubled the numer of definite cases, to 135 (40%, p<0.01). Of the 150 cased rejected by older criteria, 11 were definite, 87 were possible, and 52 were rejected by the new criteria.

Conclusion

Application of the proposed new criteria increases the number of definite diagnoses. This should be useful for more accutate diagnosis and classification of patients with suspected endocarditis and provide better entry criteria for epidemiologic studies and clinical trials.

Title	Diagnosis of 22 new cases of bartonella endocarditis.
Authors	Raoult D, Fournier PE, Drancourt M et al.
Reference	Ann Intern Med 1996;125(8):646–652.
Disease/ Pathogen	Bartonella endocarditis.
Purpose	To report the occurrence of, risk factors for, and clinical feature of bartonella endocarditis and to evaluate the diagnostic tools available for the condition.
Design	Multicenter, case series and comparison with past series.
Patients	22 patients from France, England, Canada, and South Africa were investigated for blood culture-negative endocarditis.
Follow-up	Titer of antibodies to bartonella species by micro-immunofluorescence assay, blood or vegetation culture, and amplifcation of bartonella DNA from valvular tissure polymerase chain reaction. Cross-absorption was done for patients with antibodies to chlamydia species.

Results   22 patients had definite endocarditis. Five were infected with bartonella quintana, 4 with Bartonella henselae, and 13 with an undetermined bartonella species. These cases were compared with the 11 previously reported cases. Of the patients with the newly reported cases, 19 had valvular surgery and 6 died. Nine were homeless, 11 were alcoholic, 4 owned cats and 13 had pre-existing valvular heart disease. Bartonella species caused 3% of the cases of endocarditis seen in the three study centers. The patients with these cases could have previously received a diagnosis of chlamycial endocarditis because of apparently high levels of cross-reacting antibodies to chlamydia species.

Conclusion   Bartonella species are an important cause of blood culture-negative endocarditis and can be identified by culture, serologic studies, or molecular biology techniques. Alcoholism and homelessness without previous valvular heart disease are risk factor for B. quintana infection, but not for infection with bartonella species.

1. Syndromes

h. Erythema Migrans

Azithromycin Compared with Amoxicillin in the Treatment of Erythema Migrans: A Double Blind, Randomized, Controlled Trial.

Title	Azithromycin compared with amoxicillin in the treatment of erythema migrans: A double blind, randomized, controlled trial.
Authors	Luft BJ, Dattwyler RJ, Johnson RC, et al.
Reference	Ann Intern Med 1996;124:785–791.
Disease/ Pathogen	Erythema migrans.
Purpose	To determine whether azithromycin or amoxicillin is more efficacious for the treatment of erythema migrans skin lesions, which are characteristic of Lyme disease.
Design	Randomized, double blind, controlled, multicenter study.
Patients	246 adult patients with erythema migrans lesions at least 5 cm in diameter were enrolled and were stratified by the presence of flu-like symptoms (such as fever, chills, headache, malaise, fatigue, arthralgias, and myalgias) before randomization.
Follow-up	180 days.
Treatment/ prophylaxis regimen	Oral treatment with either amoxicillin, 500 mg three times daily for 20 days, or azithromycin, 500 mg once daily for 7 days. Patients who received azithromycin also received a dummy placebo so that the dosing schedules were identical.

Azithromycin Compared with Amoxicillin in the Treatment of Erythema Migrans: A Double Blind, Randomized, Controlled Trial.

(continued)

Results   Of 217 evaluable patients, those treated with amoxicillin were significantly more likely than those treated with azithromycin to achieve complete resolution of disease at day 20, the end of therapy (88% compared with 76%; p=0.024). More azithromycin recipients (16%) than amoxicillin recipients (4%) had relapse (p=0.005). A partial response at day 20 was highly predictive of relapse (27% of partial responders had relapse compared with 6% of complete responders; p<0.001). For patients treated with azithromycin, development of an antibody response increased the possibility of achieving a complete response (81% of seropositive patients achieved a complete response, compared with 60% of seronegative patients; p=0.043). Patients with multiple erythema migrans lesions were more likely than patients with single erythema migrans lesions (p<0.001) to have a positive antibody titer at baseline (63% compared with 17%, for IgM; 39% compared with 16% for IgG). Fifty-seven percent of patients who had relapse were seronegative at the time of relapse.

Conclusion   A 20-day course of amoxicillin was found to be an effective therapeutic regimen for erythema migrans. Most patients were seronegative for borrelia burgdorferi at the time of presentation with erythema migrans (65%) and at the time of relapse (57%).

1. Syndromes

i. Fever of Unknown Origin

Clinical Value of Gallium-67 Scintigraphy in Evaluation of Fever of Unknown Origin

Title	Clinical value of gallium-67 scintigraphy in evaluation of fever of unknown origin.
Authors	Knockaert DC, Mortelmans LA, De Roo MC, et al.
Reference	Clin Infect Dis 1994;18(4):601–605.
Disease/ Pathogen	Fever of unknown origin.
Purpose	To describe the diagnostic contribution of gallium-67 scintigraphy in fevers of unknown origin (FUO).
Design	Gallium scintigraphy screening in a university hospital over a 9-year period.
Patients	145 cases of fever of unknown origin.
Results	A final diagnosis was established in 99 (68%) of the 145 cases. Sixty-three scans (43%) were normal, and 82 (57%) were abnormal; only 42 of the abnormal scans (29% of the total number of scans) were considered helpful in diagnosis. Thus, 49% of the abnormal scans were considered noncontributory to the diagnosis. In the same population, 15 (6%) of 266 ultrasonograms and 32 (14%) of 233 computed tomograms were helpful in diagnosis.
Conclusion	The authors conclude that gallium scintigraphy remains a valuable screening tool in the investigation of FUO: It yielded diagnostic information in 29% of cases in which the probability of a definitive diagnosis was only 68%. The authors suggest the use of gallium scintigraphy as a second-step (as opposed to a last-resort) procedure in the evaluation of FUO.

1. Syndromes

j. Gastroenteritis

Empirical Treatment of Severe Acute Community-Acquired Gastroenteritis with Ciprofloxacin

Title	Empirical treatment of severe acute community-acquired gastroenteritis with ciprofloxacin.
Authors	Dryden MS, Gabb RJ, Wright SK.
Reference	Clin Infect Dis 1996;22(6):1019–1025.
Disease/ Pathogen	Community-acquired gastroenteritis.
Purpose	Randomized controlled trial.
Design	To determine whether empirical treatment of severe acute community-acquired gastroenteritis (four fluid stools per day for >3 days) with ciprofloxacin reduces the duration of diarrhea and other symptoms and to determine what effect ciprofloxacin has on the duration of long-term fecal carriage of gastrointestinal pathogens.
Patients	A total of 173 patients were recruited for the study.
Follow-up	Fecal samples were collected before treatment and regularly after treatment to determine the duration of carriage of gastrointestinal pathogens. Antibiotic susceptibility tests were performed, and the minimum inhibitory concentrations (MICs) of ciprofloxacin were determined.
Treatment/ prophylaxis regimen	Patients received either ciprofloxacin (500 mg b.i.d.) or placebo for 5 days, during which time they recorded the duration of diarrhea and other symptoms (fever, abdominal pain, vomiting, and myalgia).

Results

A significant reduction in the duration of diarrhea and other symptoms was observed after treatment, regardless of whether a pathogen was detected (p=0.0001). Treatment failure occurred in 3 of 81 patients in the ciprofloxacin group and 17 of 81 patients in the placebo group. Significant pathogens were detected in 87% of patients, 85.5% of whom had cleared the pathogen at the end of treatment with ciprofloxacin, as compared with 34% who received placebo. Six weeks after treatment, there was no difference between the two groups in terms of the pathogen carriage rate (12%). Treatment with ciprofloxacin did not prolong carriage. High-level resistance to ciprofloxacin (MIC, >32 mg/L) was detected in three strains (4%) of campylobacter species.

Conclusion

Ciprofloxacin appears to be effective in reducing the duration of diarrhea and in the early clearance of pathogens.

1. Syndromes

k. Guillain-Barré Syndrome

Randomised Trial of Plasma Exchange, Intravenous Immunoglobulin, and Combined Treatments in Guillain-Barré Syndrome

Title	Randomised trial of plasma exchange, intravenous immunoglobulin, and combined treatments in Guillain-Barré syndrome.
Reference	Lancet 1997;349:225–230.
Disease/ Pathogen	Guillain-Barré syndrome.
Purpose	We compared plasma exchange (PE) with intravenous immunoglobulin (IVIg), and with a combined regimen of PE followed by IVIg, in an international, multicenter, randomised trial of 383 adult patients with Guillain-Barre syndrome.
Design	Randomised, multicenter trial.
Patients	383 adult patients with Guillain-Barré syndrome. The inclusion criteria were severe disease (aid needed for walking) and onset of neuropathic symptoms within the previous 14 days.
Follow-up	Patients were followed up for 48 weeks.
Treatment/ prophylaxis regimen	Patients were randomly assigned PE (five 50 mL/kg exchanges over 8-13 days), IVIg (Sandoglobulin, 0.4 g/kg daily for 5 days), or the PE course immediately followed by the IVIg course.

Randomised Trial of Plasma Exchange, Intravenous Immunoglobulin, and Combined Treatments in Guillain-Barré Syndrome

(continued)

Results	Four patients were excluded because they did not meet the randomisation criteria. All the remaining 379 patients were assessed for the major outcome criterion-change on a seven-point disability grade scale by an observer unaware of treatment assignment, 4 weeks after randomisation. At that time, the mean improvement was 0.9 (SD 1.3) in the 121 PE group patients, 0.8 (1.3) in the 130 IVIg group patients, and 1.1 (1.4) in the 128 patients who received both treatments (intention-to-treat analysis). None of the differences between the groups for this major outcome criterion was significant. The difference between PE alone and IVIg alone was so small that a 0.5 grade difference was excluded at the 95% level of confidence. There was no significant difference between any of the treatment groups in the secondary outcome measures: Time to recovery of unaided walking, time to discontinuation of ventilation, and trend describing the recovery from disability up to 48 weeks. There was a non-significant trend toward a more favorable outcome on some outcome measures with combined treatment.
Conclusion	In treatment of severe Guillain-Barré syndrome during the first 2 weeks after onset of neuropathic symptoms, PE and IVIg had equivalent efficacy. The combination of PE with IVIg did not confer a significant advantage.

1. Syndromes

1. Hemolytic-Uremic Syndrome

Improved Survival in Thrombotic Thrombocytopenic Purpura-Hemolytic Uremic Syndrome: Clinical Experience in 108 Patients

Title	Improved survival in thrombotic thrombocytopenic pur-pura-hemolytic uremic syndrome. Clinical experience in 108 patients.
Authors	Bell WR, Braine HG, Ness PM, et al.
Reference	New Engl J Med 1991;325:398–403.
Disease/ Pathogen	Hemolytic uremic syndrome.
Purpose	To determine the efficacy of treatment protocols for hemolytic uremic syndrome.
Patients	108 patients with hemolytic uremic syndrome.
Treatment/ prophylaxis regimen	Treatment regimens included 200 mg of prednisone a day, for patients with minimal symptoms and no central nervous system symptoms, and prednisone plus plasma exchange, for patients with rapid clinical deterioration who did not improve after 48 hours of prednisone alone, and for patients presenting with central nervous system symptoms and a rapidly declining hematocrit values and platelet counts.

*Improved Survival in Thrombotic Thrombocytopenic
Purpura-Hemolytic Uremic Syndrome:
Clinical Experience in 108 Patients*

(continued)

Results	A total of 108 patients were treated, and 91% survived. Prednisone alone was judged to be effective in 30 patients with mild thrombotic thrombocytompenic purpura-hemolytic uremic syndrome (TTP-HUS) (two relapses and two deaths). Plasma exchange plus prednisone was given to 78 patients with complicated TTP-HUS, resulting in 67 relapses and 8 deaths. Relapses occurred in 22 of 36 patients given maintenance plasma infusions. Neither splenectomy nor treatment with aspirin and dipyridamole was effective in those with a poor response to plasma exchange. None of the 71 patients tested had positive cultures for O157:H7 Escherichia coli. Nine percent of the patients were pregnant, and none gave birth to infants with TTP-HUS.
Conclusion	Effective treatment with 91% survival is available for patients with TTP-HUS.

1. Syndromes
m. Hepatitis

Efficacy of Hepatitis A Vaccine in Prevention of Secondary Hepatitis A Infection: A Randomised Trial.

Title	Efficacy of hepatitis A vaccine in prevention of secondary hepatitis A infection: A randomised trial.
Authors	Sagliocca L, Amoroso P, Stroffolini T, et al.
Reference	Lancet 1999;353:1136–1139.
Disease/ Pathogen	Hepatitis A.
Purpose	To investigate the use of hepatitis A vaccine to prevent secondary infections with hepatitis A virus (HAV).
Design	Randomised controlled trial.
Patients	Household contacts of people with sporadic HAV infection.
Follow-up	45 days.
Treatment/ prophylaxis regimen	Households (index cases and contacts) were randomly assigned to the vaccine group or unvaccinated group, according to the study week in which they were enrolled. All household contacts in the vaccine group received vaccination at the time of entry to the study.
Results	During 45 days of follow-up, secondary infection had occurred in 10 (13.3%) of 75 households (two families had two cases each) in the untreated group and in two (2.8%) of 71 households in the vaccine group. The protective efficacy of the vaccine was 79% (95% Confidence Interval [CI] 7–95). The number of secondary infections among household contacts was 12 (5.8%) of 207 in the unvaccinated group, and two (1%) of 197 in the vaccinated group. Therefore, 18 individuals needed to be vaccinated to prevent one secondary infection.

Conclusion   Hepatitis A vaccine is effective in the prevention of secondary infection of HAV and should be recommended for household contacts of primary cases of HAV infection.

Randomised Trial of Interferon Alpha2b Plus Ribavirin for 48 Weeks or for 24 Weeks Vs Interferon Alpha2b Plus Placebo for 48 Weeks for Treatment of Chronic Infection with Hepatitis C Virus

Title	Randomised trial of interferon alpha2b plus ribavirin for 48 weeks or for 24 weeks vs interferon alpha2b plus placebo for 48 weeks for treatment of chronic infection with hepatitis C virus.
Authors	Poynard T, Marcellin P, Lee SS, et al.
Reference	Lancet 1998;352:1426–1432.
Disease/ Pathogen	Hepatitis C.
Purpose	The aim of this study was to compare the efficacy and safety of interferon alpha2b in combination with oral ribavirin with interferon alone, for treatment of chronic infection with hepatitis C virus (HCV).
Design	Randomised, placebo controlled.
Patients	832 patients aged 18 years or more with chronic HCV who had not been treated with interferon or ribavirin.
Follow-up	All patients were assessed for safety, tolerance, and efficacy at the end of weeks 1, 2, 4, 6, and 8, and every 4 weeks during treatment. After treatment was completed, patients were followed up on weeks 4, 8, 12, and 24. The primary end-point was loss of detectable HCV-RNA (serum HCV-ribonucleic acid <100 copies/mL) at week 24 after treatment.

Randomised Trial of Interferon Alpha2b Plus Ribavirin for 48 Weeks or for 24 Weeks Vs Interferon Alpha2b Plus Placebo for 48 Weeks for Treatment of Chronic Infection with Hepatitis C Virus

(continued)

Treatment/ prophylaxis regimen	3 mega units (MU) interferon alpha2b three times a week plus 1000–1200 mg ribavirin per day for 48 weeks; 3 MU interferon alpha2b three times a week plus 1000–1200 mg ribavirin per day for 24 weeks; or 3 MU interferon alpha2b three times a week and placebo for 48 weeks.
Results	Sustained virological response at 24 weeks after treatment was found in 119 (43%) of the 277 patients treated for 48 weeks with the combination regimen, 97 (35%) of the 277 patients treated for 24 weeks with the combination regimen (p=0.055), and 53 (19%) of the 278 patients treated for 48 weeks with interferon alone (p<0.001 vs both combination regimens, intention-to-treat analysis). Logistic regression identified five independent factors significantly associated with response: Genotype 2 or 3, viral load less than 2 million copies/mL, age 40 years or less, minimal fibrosis stage, and female sex. Among patients with fewer than three of these factors the odds ratio of sustained response was 2.6 (95% confidence interval 1.4–4.8; p=0.002) for the 48 week combination regimen compared with 24 weeks of the combination regimen. Discontinuation of therapy for adverse events was more frequent with combination (19%) and monotherapy (13%) given for 48 weeks than combination therapy given for 24 weeks (8%).
Conclusion	An interferon alpha2b plus ribavirin combination is more effective than 48 weeks of interferon alpha2b monotherapy, and has an acceptable safety profile. Patients with few favorable factors benefit more from extending the duration of combination therapy to 48 weeks.

Randomised, Double Blind, Placebo Controlled Trial of Interferon Alpha-2b With and Without Ribavirin for Chronic Hepatitis C

Title	Randomised, double blind, placebo controlled trial of interferon alpha-2b with and without ribavirin for chronic hepatitis C.
Authors	Reichard O, Norkrans G, Fryden A, et al.
Reference	Lancet 1998;351:83–87.
Disease/ Pathogen	Hepatitis C.
Purpose	To investigate the biochemical and virological responses and safety of treatment with interferon alpha-2b and ribavirin, compared with interferon alpha-2b alone.
Design	Randomised, double blind, placebo controlled.
Patients	100 pateints with hepatitis C.
Follow-up	Patients were followed for 24 weeks after the 24 weeks of therapy, and then one-year after the active treatment stopped. The primary end-point was the sustained virological response, defined as no detectable HCV-RNA by polymerase chain reaction at both week 24 and week 48.
Treatment/ prophylaxis regimen	Patients were randomly assigned to treatment with interferon alpha-2b (3 mega units three times a week) in combination with ribavirin (1000 or 1200 mg per day) or placebo for 24 weeks.

***Randomised, Double Blind, Placebo Controlled Trial of
Interferon Alpha-2b With and Without Ribavirin for
Chronic Hepatitis C***

(continued)

Results 18 (36%) of the 50 patients in the interferon alpha-2b and
ribavirin group had a sustained virological response, compared with nine (18%) of the 50 patients in the interferon
alpha-2b and placebo group (p=0.047). At the 1-year follow-up, the proportion of patients with a virological
response was greater in the interferon alpha-2b and ribavirin group, than the interferon alpha-2b and placebo
group (42% vs 20%, p=0.03), respectively. More patients
with baseline HCV-RNA concentrations greater than 3 x
10(6) genome equivalents (Eq) per mL had a sustained
response with interferon alpha-2b and ribavirin than with
interferon alpha-2b and placebo (12/29 vs 1/26, p=0.009),
whereas the sustained response did not differ between
the two treatment groups for HCV-RNA amounts less than
3 x 10(6) Eq per mL (6/21 vs 8/24, p=0.67), respectively.

Conclusion More patients with chronic hepatitis C have a sustained
virological response with interferon alpha-2b and ribavirin than with only interferon alpha-2b treatment. We
suggest that patients with high HCV-RNA loads should be
treated with interferon alpha-2b and ribavirin.

A Controlled Study of Hepatitis C Transmission by Organ Transplantation

Title	A controlled study of hepatitis C transmission by organ transplantation.
Authors	Pereira BJ, Wright TL, Schmid CH, et al.
Reference	Lancet 1995;345:484–487.
Disease/ Pathogen	Hepatitis C.
Purpose	To determine the outcomes of organ recipients who receive organs from anti-hepatitis C virus (HCV) positive and negative donors.
Design	Clinical records were reviewed and recipient sera were tested for anti-HCV with a second-generation enzyme-linked immunosorbent assay (ELISA), and HCV-RNA was tested for by polymerase chain reaction.
Patients	29 recipients who received organs from anti-HCV positive donors were the study group. 37 donors were randomly selected from 703 ELISA1-negative cadaver organ donors. 74 recipients of organs from these 37 donors were the control group.
Follow-up	Median post-transplant follow-up was 42 and 49 months for study and control groups, respectively.

Results

Post-transplantation prevalence of anti-HCV and HCV-RNA was 67% and 96% among recipients from anti-HCV-positive donors, and 20% and 18% among recipients from anti-HCV-negative donors (p<0.001), respectively. Post-transplantation non-A, non-B hepatitis, graft loss, and death were observed in 55%, 52%, and 31% among recipients of organs from anti-HCV-positive donors, and 16%, 53%, and 33% among recipients from anti-HCV-negative donors. In a proportional hazards model, the relative risks for non-A, non-B hepatitis, graft loss, and death among recipients from anti-HCV-positive donors were 4.37 (95% confidence interval 1.97–9.70), 0.93 (0.51–1.70), and 0.89 (0.41–1.93).

Conclusion

Transmission of HCV infection by organ transplantation increased the risk of liver disease among recipients. However, after 3.5 years, donor HCV infection did not adversely affect patient survival or graft survival.

Title	A 1-year trial of lamivudine for chronic hepatitis B.
Authors	Lai CL, Chien RN, Leung NWY, et al.
Reference	N Engl J Med 1998;339:61–68.
Disease/ Pathogen	Hepatitis B.
Purpose	To determine whether a longer duration of viral suppression (one year) would result in improved histologic findings, higher hepatitis B e antigen (HBeAg) seroconversion rates, or both, in patients with chronic hepatitis B.
Design	Randomized, double blind, placebo controlled, multicenter.
Patients	A total of 358 Chinese patients were randomly assigned to receive 25 mg of lamivudine (142 patients), 100 mg of lamivudine (143), or placebo (73).
Follow-up	The primary end-point was a reduction of at least two points in the Knodell necro-inflammatory score.
Treatment/ prophylaxis regimen	The patients were randomly assigned to receive 25 mg of lamivudine, 100 mg of lamivudine, or placebo, given orally once a day for 12 months (ratio of random assignments to the three groups, 2:2:1).

Results

Hepatic necro-inflammatory activity improved by two points or more in 56% of the patients receiving 100 mg of lamivudine, 49% of those receiving 25 mg of lamivudine, and 25% of those receiving placebo ($p<0.001$ and $p=0.001$, respectively, for the comparisons of lamivudine treatment with placebo). Necro-inflammatory activity worsened in 7% of the patients receiving 100 mg of lamivudine, 8% of those receiving 25 mg, and 26% of those receiving placebo. The 100-mg dose of lamivudine was associated with a reduced progression of fibrosis ($p=0.01$ for the comparison with placebo) and with the highest rate of HBeAg seroconversion (loss of HbeAg, development of antibody to HbeAg, and undetectable HBV DNA) (16%), the greatest suppression of HBV DNA (98% reduction at week 52, as compared with the baseline value), and the highest rate of sustained normalization of alanine aminotransferase levels (72%). 96% of the patients completed the study. The incidence of adverse events was similar in all groups, and there were few serious events.

Conclusion

In a 1-year study, lamivudine was associated with substantial histologic improvement in many patients with chronic hepatitis B. A daily dose of 100 mg was more effective than a daily dose of 25 mg.

Interferon Alfa-2b Alone or in Combination with Ribavirin as Initial Treatment for Chronic Hepatitis C

Title	Interferon alfa-2b alone or in combination with ribavirin as initial treatment for chronic hepatitis C.
Authors	McHutchison JG, Gordon SC, Schiff ER, et al.
Reference	N Engl J Med 1998;339:1485–1492.
Disease/ Pathogen	Hepatitis C.
Purpose	To compare the safety and efficacy of interferon alone and in combination with ribavirin for the initial treatment of chronic hepatitis C virus (HCV) and to determine the optimal duration of combination therapy.
Design	Randomized, double blind, placebo controlled, multicenter.
Patients	912 patients with chronic hepatitis C randomly assigned to one of four treatment groups, which were balanced for the presence or absence of cirrhosis, pretreatment serum HCV-ribonucleic acid level (RNA), and HCV genotype.
Follow-up	24 and 48 weeks.
Treatment/ prophylaxis regimen	Interferon alfa-2b was given subcutaneously in a dose of 3 million units three times per week, and ribavirin (or matched placebo) was administered orally twice a day at a total daily dose of 1000 mg for patients who weighed 75 kg or less and 1200 mg for those who weighed more than 75 kg.

Results

The rate of sustained virologic response (defined as an undetectable serum HCV-RNA level 24 weeks after treatment was completed) was higher among patients who received combination therapy for either 24 weeks (70 of 228 patients, 31%), or 48 weeks (87 of 228 patients, 38%) than among patients who received interferon alone for either 24 weeks (13 of 231 patients, 6%) or 48 weeks (29 of 225 patients, 13%) (p<0.001 for the comparison of interferon alone with both 24 weeks and 48 weeks of combination treatment). Among patients with HCV genotype 1 infection, the best response occurred in those who were treated for 48 weeks with interferon and ribavirin. Histologic improvement was more common in patients who were treated with combination therapy for either 24 weeks (57%) or 48 weeks (61%) than in those who were treated with interferon alone for either 24 weeks (44%) or 48 weeks (41%). The drug doses had to be reduced and treatment discontinued more often in patients who were treated with combination therapy.

Conclusion

In patients with chronic hepatitis C, initial therapy with interferon and ribavirin was more effective than treatment with interferon alone.

Ribavirin as Therapy for Chronic Hepatitis C:
A Randomized, Double Blind, Placebo Controlled Trial.

Title	Ribavirin as therapy for chronic hepatitis C: A randomized, double blind, placebo controlled trial.
Authors	Di Bisceglie AM, Conjeevaram HS, Fried MW, et al.
Reference	Ann Inter Med 1995;123:897–903.
Disease/ Pathogen	Hepatitis C.
Purpose	To evaluate ribavirin, an oral antiviral agent, as therapy for chronic hepatitis C.
Design	Randomized, double blind, placebo controlled study.
Patients	29 patients with chronic hepatitis C.
Follow-up	6 months.
Treatment/ prophylaxis regimen	29 patients with chronic hepatitis C who received oral ribavirin (600 mg twice daily) for 12 months and 29 controls with chronic hepatitis C who received placebo for 12 months.

Ribavirin as Therapy for Chronic Hepatitis C:
A Randomized, Double Blind, Placebo Controlled Trial.

(continued)

Results	Patients treated with ribavirin had a prompt decrease in serum aminotransferase levels (54% overall) compared with levels before treatment and levels in controls (5% decrease). Serum aminotransferase levels became normal or nearly normal in 10 patients treated with ribavirin (35% [95% confidence interval [CI] 18%-54%]) but in no controls (0% [CI 0%-12%]). Aminotransferase levels remained normal in only two patients after ribavirin therapy was discontinued (7% [CI, 1%-23%]). Serum HCV-ribonucleic acid levels did not change during or after therapy. Liver biopsy specimens showed a decrease in hepatic inflammation and necrosis among ribavirin-treated patients whose aminotransferase levels became normal.
Conclusion	Ribavirin has beneficial effects on serum aminotransferase levels and histologic findings in the liver in patients with chronic hepatitis C, but these effects are not accompanied by changes in HCV-RNA levels and are not sustained when ribavirin therapy is discontinued. Thus, ribavirin alone for periods as long as 12 months is unlikely to be of value as therapy for chronic hepatitis C.

Decrease in Serum Hepatitis C Viral RNA During Alpha-Interferon Therapy for Chronic Hepatitis C

Title	Decrease in serum hepatitis C viral RNA during alpha-interferon therapy for chronic hepatitis C.
Authors	Shindo M, Di Bisceglie AM, Cheung L, et al.
Reference	Ann Intern Med 1991;115:700–704.
Disease/ Pathogen	Hepatitis C.
Purpose	To assess the effect of alpha-interferon therapy on hepatitis C viral ribonucleic acid (RNA) in serum of patients with chronic hepatitis C.
Design	Retrospective testing for hepatitis C viral (HCV) RNA and antibody to the hepatitis C virus (anti-HCV) of stored serum samples from a randomized, double blind, placebo controlled trial of alpha-interferon therapy.
Patients	41 patients with chronic non-A, non-B hepatitis were entered in this trial.
Follow-up	Samples were tested for anti-HCV by enzyme-linked immunosorbent assay. Hepatitis C viral RNA was detected in serum using the polymerase chain reaction. Titers of both antibody and RNA were determined by serial end-point dilution.
Treatment/ prophylaxis regimen	Twenty-one patients were treated with alpha-interferon, and 20 patients were treated with placebo for 6 months. Seventeen placebo recipients were then treated with alpha-interferon for up to 1 year.

Results

At entry into the trial, 37 (90%) of 41 patients had anti-HCV, and 39 (95%) had HCV-RNA in serum. Anti-HCV titers decreased slightly with treatment. Serum levels of HCV RNA decreased in all patients who responded to alpha-interferon therapy with improvements in serum aminotransferases; in 17 of 21 responders (81%; 95% confidence interval [CI] 58%–95%) HCV-RNA became undetectable. In contrast, in only 2 of 16 (12%; CI 2%–38%) patients who did not respond to treatment did HCV-RNA become undetectable. In 19 patients treated during the preliminary 6-month period with placebo, HCV-RNA remained detectable. Finally, in the 11 patients who relapsed when treatment was stopped, HCV RNA reappeared in the serum, but in four of seven patients with a sustained improvement in serum aminotransferases, HCV-RNA remained undetectable.

Conclusion

These results indicate that the clinical and serum biochemical response to alpha-interferon in chronic hepatitis C is associated with a loss of detectable HCV genome from serum.

1. Syndromes

n. Onychomycosis

Double Blind, Randomized Study of Continuous Terbinafine Compared with Intermittent Itraconazole in Treatment of Toenail Onychomycosis

Title	Double blind, randomized study of continuous terbinafine compared with intermittent itraconazole in treatment of toenail onychomycosis.
Authors	Evans EG, Sigurgeirsson B.
Reference	BMJ 1999;318(7190):1031–1035.
Disease/ Pathogen	Dermatophyte onychomycosis.
Purpose	To compare the efficacy and safety of continuous terbinafine with intermittent itraconazole in the treatment of toenail onychomycosis.
Design	Prospective, randomized, double blind, double dummy, multicenter, parallel group study lasting 72 weeks.
Patients	496 patients aged 18 to 75 years with a clinical and mycological diagnosis of dermatophyte onychomycosis of the toenail.
Follow-up	Assessment of primary efficacy at week 72 was mycological cure, defined as negative results on microscopy and culture of samples from the target toenail.
Treatment/ prophylaxis regimen	Study patients were randomly divided into four parallel groups to receive either terbinafine 250 mg a day for 12 or 16 weeks (groups T12 and T16) or itraconazole 400 mg a day for 1 week in every 4 weeks for 12 or 16 weeks (groups I3 and I4).

*Double Blind, Randomized Study of Continuous Terbinafine
Compared with Intermittent Itraconazole in Treatment
of Toenail Onychomycosis*

(continued)

Results   At week 72, the mycological cure rates were 75.7%
                (81/107) in the T12 group and 80. 8% (80/99) in the T16
                group compared, with 38.3% (41/107) in the I3 group and
                49.1% (53/108) in the I4 group. All comparisons (T12 vs
                I3, T12 vs I4, T16 vs I3, T16 vs I4) showed significantly
                higher cure rates in the terbinafine groups (all p<0.0001).
                Also, all secondary clinical outcome measures were sig-
                nificantly in favor of terbinafine at week 72. There were
                no differences in the number or type of adverse events
                recorded in the terbinafine or itraconazole groups.

Conclusion   Continuous terbinafine is significantly more effective than
                intermittent itraconazole in the treatment of patients with
                toenail onychomycosis.

1. Syndromes

o. Pancreatitis

Title	Early antibiotic treatment in acute necrotising pancreatitis.
Authors	Sainio V, Kemppainen E, Puolakkainen P, et al.
Reference	Lancet 1995;346:663–667.
Disease/ Pathogen	Pancreatitis.
Purpose	To determine the effect of early antibiotic treatment on the outcome of alcohol-induced necrotizing pancreatitis.
Design	Randomized trial.
Patients	60 consecutive patients with alcohol-induced necrotising pancreatitis. The inclusion criteria were C-reactive protein concentration above 120 mg/L within 48 h of admission, and low enhancement (<30 Hounsfield units) on contrast-enhanced computed tomography.
Treatment/ prophylaxis regimen	30 patients were assigned cefuroxime (4.5 g/day intravenously) from admission. In the second group, no antibiotic treatment was given until clinical or microbiologically verified infection or after a secondary rise in C-reactive protein.

(continued)

Results	There were more infectious complications in the non-antibiotic than in the antibiotic group (mean per patient 1.8 vs 1, p=0.01). The most common cause of sepsis was staphylococcus epidermidis; positive cultures were obtained from pancreatic necrosis or the central venous line in 14 of 18 patients with suspected but blood-culture-negative sepsis. Mortality was higher in the non-antibiotic group (seven vs one in the antibiotic group; p=0.03). Four of the eight patients who died had cultures from pancreatic necrosis positive for staphylococcus epidermidis.
Conclusion	The authors conclude that cefuroxime given early in necrotising pancreatitis is beneficial and may reduce mortality, probably by decreasing the frequency of sepsis.

Title	Differential prognosis of gram-negative vs gram-positive infected and sterile pancreatic necrosis: Results of a randomized trial in patients with severe acute pancreatitis treated with adjuvant selective decontamination.
Authors	Luiten EJ, Hop WC, Lange JF, et al.
Reference	Clin Infect Dis 1997;25(4):811–816.
Disease/ Pathogen	Pancreatitis.
Purpose	To compare the differential prognosis of gram-negative vs gram-positive and sterile pancreatic necrosis in patients treated with adjuvant selective decontamination.
Design	Randomized, multicenter trial.
Patients	102 patients with severe acute pancreatitis.
Treatment/ prophylaxis regimen	Patients treated with or without adjuvant selective decontamination were analyzed with regard to the bacteriologic status of (peri)pancreatic necrosis.

Differential Prognosis of Gram-Negative Vs Gram-Positive Infected and Sterile Pancreatic Necrosis: Results of a Randomized Trial in Patients with Severe Acute Pancreatitis Treated with Adjuvant Selective Decontamination.

(continued)

Results	The incidence of gram-negative pancreatic infection was significantly reduced in patients treated with selective decontamination (p=0.004). Once such an infection develops, mortality increases 15-fold (p<0.001) in comparison with that for patients with sterile necrosis. Among patients in whom only gram-positive infection of pancreatic necrosis was found, there was no significant increase in mortality. These results were similar in both treatment groups. In addition, the hospital stay was significantly longer in cases of gram-negative infected necrosis. The incidence of gram-positive infected necrosis in patients treated with selective decontamination did not increase.
Conclusion	Gram-negative pancreatic infection can be prevented with adjuvant selective decontamination, thereby reducing mortality among patients with severe acute pancreatitis.

1. Syndromes

p. Pelvic Inflammatory Disease

Comparison of Three Regimens Recommended by the Centers for Disease Control and Prevention for the Treatment of Women Hospitalized with Acute Pelvic Inflammatory Disease

Title	Comparison of three regimens recommended by the Centers for Disease Control and Prevention for the treatment of women hospitalized with acute pelvic inflammatory disease.
Authors	Hemsell DL, Little BB, Faro S, et al.
Reference	Clin Infect Dis 1994;19(4):720–727.
Disease/ Pathogen	Pelvic inflammatory disease (PID).
Purpose	To compare the efficacy and safety of three regimens recommended by the Centers for Disease Control and Prevention (CDC) for the treatment of women hospitalized for the treatment of acute pelvic inflammatory disease.
Design	Prospective, open label, multicenter, clinical trial. A severity score was used for objective comparison of the degree of illness before and after therapy.
Patients	292 women with pelvic inflammatory disease.
Follow-up	Response to inpatient therapy.
Treatment/ prophylaxis regimen	Women were randomly assigned (in a 1:1:1 ratio) to treatment with cefoxitin plus doxycycline, clindamycin plus gentamicin, or cefotetan plus doxycycline.

Comparison of Three Regimens Recommended by the Centers for Disease Control and Prevention for the Treatment of Women Hospitalized with Acute Pelvic Inflammatory Disease

(continued)

Results	Two hundred seventy-five (94.2%) of 292 evaluable women required no alteration in therapeutic regimen. The three regimens produced almost identical cure rates. No serious adverse clinical or laboratory events were observed.
Conclusion	The authors conclude the three regimens recommended by the CDC for inpatient therapy of acute PID were similarly effective and safe.

A Multicenter Study Comparing Intravenous Meropenem with Clindamycin Plus Gentamicin for the Treatment of Acute Gynecologic and Obstetric Pelvic Infections in Hospitalized Women

Title	A multicenter study comparing intravenous meropenem with clindamycin plus gentamicin for the treatment of acute gynecologic and obstetric pelvic infections in hospitalized women.
Authors	Hemsell DL, Martens MG, Faro S, et al.
Reference	Clin Infect Dis 1997;24 Suppl 2:S222–S230.
Disease/ Pathogen	Gynecologic and obstetric pelvic infections.
Purpose	To compare the efficacy and safety of meropenem with the efficacy and safety of clindamycin plus gentamicin in the treatment of patients with acute gynecologic and obstetric pelvic infections.
Design	Multicenter, prospective clinical trial.
Patients	515 hospitalized patients with acute gynecologic and obstetric pelvic infections.
Treatment/ prophylaxis regimen	Patients received either meropenem or clindamycin plus gentamicin.

A Multicenter Study Comparing Intravenous Meropenem with Clindamycin Plus Gentamicin for the Treatment of Acute Gynecologic and Obstetric Pelvic Infections in Hospitalized Women

(continued)

Results	At the end of treatment, the rates of satisfactory clinical and bacteriologic response were high (88%) in both treatment groups: The rates of response were 90% for the meropenem group and 86% for the clindamycin/gentamicin group. No serious adverse events occurred. The most frequently reported drug-related adverse clinical events in the meropenem group were nausea and injection-site reactions (>1% of patients), and the most common drug-related laboratory abnormality was thrombocythemia. Similar patterns of adverse events occurred in the clindamycin/gentamicin group. However, the incidence of diarrhea and eosinophilia was higher in this group.
Conclusion	This trial demonstrated that meropenem is an effective and safe alternative to the combination of clindamycin plus gentamicin for the treatment of women with acute gynecologic and obstetric pelvic infections.

Oral Clindamycin and Ciprofloxacin Vs Intramuscular Ceftriaxone and Oral Doxycycline in the Treatment of Mild-to-Moderate Pelvic Inflammatory Disease in Outpatients

Title	Oral clindamycin and ciprofloxacin vs intramuscular ceftriaxone and oral doxycycline in the treatment of mild-to-moderate pelvic inflammatory disease in outpatients.
Authors	Arredondo JL, Diaz V, Gaitan H, et al.
Reference	Clin Infect Dis 1997;24(2):170–178.
Disease/ Pathogen	Pelvic inflammatory disease.
Purpose	To compare the safety and efficacy of clindamycin and ciprofloxacin vs ceftriaxone and doxycycline in the treatment of outpatients with mild-to-moderate pelvic inflammatory disease (PID) diagnosed by laparoscopy.
Design	Multicenter, prospective, double blind study.
Patients	Of the 138 patients enrolled, 131 were evaluable for efficacy.
Treatment/ prophylaxis regimen	Patients received either oral clindamycin and ciprofloxacin or intramuscular ceftriaxone and doxycycline.

Oral Clindamycin and Ciprofloxacin Vs Intramuscular Ceftriaxone and Oral Doxycycline in the Treatment of Mild-to-Moderate Pelvic Inflammatory Disease in Outpatients

(continued)

Results	Samples taken from the endocervix, endometrium, and abdominal cavity before treatment, and from the endocervix after treatment, were cultured for aerobes, anaerobes, Neisseria gonorrhoeae, and Chlamydia trachomatis. The most prevalent bacteria were streptococci, staphylococci, and Escherichia coli (among aerobes) and Bacteroides species and peptostreptococci (among anaerobes). N. gonorrhoeae was present in 2% (3) of the 131 evaluable patients, and C. trachomatis was in 11% (15). The clinical cure rate was 97% in the clindamycin and ciprofloxacin group, and 95% in the ceftriaxone and doxycycline group. Side effects were similar in both groups.
Conclusion	The two regimens for the outpatient treatment of mild to moderate PID were similarly effective and safe.

1. Syndromes
q. Peritonitis

Trimethoprim-Sulfamethoxazole for the Prevention of Spontaneous Bacterial Peritonitis in Cirrhosis: A Randomized Trial.

Title	Trimethoprim-sulfamethoxazole for the prevention of spontaneous bacterial peritonitis in cirrhosis: A randomized trial.
Authors	Singh N, Gayowski T, Yu VL, et al.
Reference	Ann Intern Med 1995;122(8):595–598.
Disease/ Pathogen	Spontaneous bacterial peritonitis.
Purpose	To assess the efficacy and safety of trimethoprim-sulfamethoxazole for the prevention of spontaneous bacterial peritonitis in patients with cirrhosis and ascites.
Design	Randomized controlled trial.
Patients	60 consecutive patients with cirrhosis and ascites.
Follow-up	The median duration of follow-up for the study patients was 90 days.
Treatment/ prophylaxis regimen	Consecutive patients were randomly assigned to receive either no prophylaxis or trimethoprim-sulfamethoxazole, one double-strength tablet daily, five times a week (Monday through Friday). Patient entry was stratified by serum bilirubin (>51 micromole/L [>3 mg/dL]), ascitic fluid protein (<1 g/dL), and serum creatinine (>177 micromole/L [>2 mg/dL]) levels to ensure that high-risk patients would be similarly distributed in the two groups.

Trimethoprim-Sulfamethoxazole for the Prevention of Spontaneous Bacterial Peritonitis in Cirrhosis: A Randomized Trial

(continued)

Results	Spontaneous bacterial peritonitis or spontaneous bacteremia developed in 27% (8 of 30) of patients who did not receive prophylaxis compared with 3% (1 of 30) of patients receiving trimethoprim-sulfamethoxazole (p=0.025). Overall, infections developed in 9 of 30 patients (30%) not receiving prophylaxis and in 1 of 30 patients (3%) receiving trimethoprim-sulfamethoxazole (p=0.012). Death occurred in 6 of 30 patients (20%) who did not receive prophylaxis and in 2 of 30 patients (7%) who received trimethoprim-sulfamethoxazole (p= 0.15). Side effects—particularly hematologic toxicity—could not be attributed to trimethoprim-sulfamethoxazole in any patient.
Conclusion	Trimethoprim-sulfamethoxazole was efficacious, safe, and cost-effective for the prevention of spontaneous bacterial peritonitis in patients with cirrhosis.

1. Syndromes

r. Pneumonia

Nosocomial Pneumonia in Mechanically Ventilated Patients Receiving Antacid, Ranitidine, or Sucralfate as Prophylaxis for Stress Ulcer: A Randomized, Controlled Trial

Title	Nosocomial pneumonia in mechanically ventilated patients receiving antacid, ranitidine, or sucralfate as prophylaxis for stress ulcer: A randomized, controlled trial.
Authors	Prod'hom G, Leuenberger P, Koerfer J, et al.
Reference	Ann Intern Med 1994;120:653–662.
Disease/ Pathogen	Pneumonia.
Purpose	To assess three anti-stress ulcer prophylaxis regimens in mechanically ventilated patients for bacterial colonization, early- and late-onset nosocomial pneumonia, and gastrointestinal bleeding.
Design	Randomized controlled trial.
Patients	Consecutive eligible patients with mechanical ventilation and a nasogastric tube. Of 258 eligible patients, 244 were assessable.
Follow-up	4 days.
Treatment/ prophylaxis regimen	At intubation, patients were randomly assigned to receive one of the following: Antacid (a suspension of aluminum hydroxide and magnesium hydroxide), 20 mL every 2 hours; ranitidine, 150 mg as a continuous intravenous infusion; or sucralfate, 1 g every 4 hours.

Nosocomial Pneumonia in Mechanically Ventilated Patients Receiving Antacid, Ranitidine, or Sucralfate as Prophylaxis for Stress Ulcer: A Randomized, Controlled Trial

(continued)

Results
Of 244 assessable patients, macroscopic gastric bleeding was observed in 10%, 4%, and 6% of patients assigned to receive sucralfate, antacid, and ranitidine, respectively ($p>0.2$). The incidence of early-onset pneumonia was not statistically different among the three treatment groups ($p>0.2$). Among the 213 patients observed for more than 4 days, late-onset pneumonia was observed in 5% of the patients who received sucralfate, compared with 16% and 21% of the patients who received antacid or ranitidine, respectively ($p=0.022$). Mortality was not statistically different among the three treatment groups. Patients who received sucralfate had a lower median gastric pH ($p<0.001$), and less frequent gastric colonization, compared with the other groups ($p=0.015$). Using molecular typing, 84% of the patients with late-onset gram-negative bacillary pneumonia were found to have gastric colonization with the same bacteria before pneumonia developed.

Conclusion
Stress ulcer prophylaxis with sucralfate reduces the risk for late-onset pneumonia in ventilated patients compared with antacid or ranitidine.

The Protective Efficacy of Polyvalent Pneumococcal Polysaccharide Vaccine

Title	The protective efficacy of polyvalent pneumococcal polysaccharide vaccine.
Authors	Shapiro ED, Berg AT, Austrian R, et al.
Reference	New Engl J Med 1991;325:1453–1460.
Disease/ Pathogen	Pneumonia.
Purpose	To assess the vaccine's protective efficacy against invasive pneumococcal infections.
Design	Multicenter, hospital based, case control study.
Patients	Adults in whom Streptococcus pneumoniae was isolated from any normally sterile site.
Treatment/ prophylaxis regimen	Contacted of all providers of medical care to ascertain each subject's history of immunization with pneumococcal vaccine.

(continued)

Results

13% of the 1054 case patients, and 20% of the 1054 matched controls, had received pneumococcal vaccine (p<0.001). When vaccine was given in either its 14-valent or its 23-valent form, its aggregate protective efficacy (calculated as a percentage: 1 minus the odds ratio of having been vaccinated x 100) against infections caused by the serotypes represented in the vaccine was 56% (95% confidence interval [CI] 42%-67%; p<0.00001) for all 983 patients infected with a serotype represented in the vaccine, 61% for a subgroup of 808 immunocompetent patients (95% CI 47%-72%; p<0.00001), and 21% for a subgroup of 175 immunocompromised patients (95% CI -55%-60%; p=0.48). The vaccine was not efficacious against infections caused by serotypes not represented in the vaccine (protective efficacy, -73%; 95% CI -263%-18%; p=0.15).

Conclusion

Polyvalent pneumococcal vaccine is efficacious in preventing invasive pneumococcal infections in immunocompetent patients with indications for its administration. This vaccine should be used more widely.

Randomised Trial of 23-Valent Pneumococcal Capsular Polysaccharide Vaccine in Prevention of Pneumonia in Middle-Aged and Elderly People

Title	Randomised trial of 23-valent pneumococcal capsular polysaccharide vaccine in prevention of pneumonia in middle-aged and elderly people.
Authors	Ortqvist A, Hedlund J, Burman LA, et al.
Reference	Lancet 1998;351:399–403.
Disease/ Pathogen	Pneumonia.
Purpose	To assess the effectiveness of a 23-valent pneumococcal vaccine in the prevention of pneumococcal pneumonia and of pneumonia overall in non-immunocompromised middle-aged and elderly people.
Design	Prospective, multicenter, double blind, randomised, placebo controlled trial.
Patients	691 non-immunocompromised patients aged 50–85 years who had been treated as inpatients for community-acquired pneumonia (CAP).
Follow-up	Cox regression models were employed to estimate the relative risks of pneumonia overall, and pneumococcal pneumonia for the placebo group, compared with the vaccine group.
Treatment/ prophylaxis regimen	Patients were randomly assigned either 23-valent pneumococcal capsular polysaccharide vaccine or placebo (sodium chloride).

Randomised Trial of 23-Valent Pneumococcal Capsular Polysaccharide Vaccine in Prevention of Pneumonia in Middle-Aged and Elderly People

(continued)

Results	63 (19%) of 339 patients in the vaccine group, and 57 (16%) of 352 patients in the placebo group, developed a new pneumonia, corresponding to a relative risk over time for the placebo group, compared with the vaccine group of 0.83 (95% confidence interval [CI] 0.58–1.12, p=0.31). Pneumococcal pneumonia was diagnosed in 16 (4.5%) patients in the placebo group, and in 19 (5.6%) in the vaccine group, corresponding to a relative risk for the placebo group of 0.78 (95% CI 0.40–1.51, p=0.45). We found no difference in the death rate between the two study groups.
Conclusion	The 23-valent pneumococcal polysaccharide vaccine did not prevent pneumonia overall or pneumococcal pneumonia in middle-aged and elderly individuals.

New and Emerging Etiologies for Community-Acquired Pneumonia with Implications for Therapy: A Prospective, Multicenter Study of 359 Cases.

Title	New and emerging etiologies for community-acquired pneumonia with implications for therapy: A prospective, multicenter study of 359 cases.
Authors	Fang GD, Fine M, Orloff J, et al.
Reference	Medicine 1990;69:307–316.
Disease/ Pathogen	Pneumonia.
Purpose	To determine emerging etiologies of community-acquired pneumonia.
Design	Prospective, multicenter study.
Patients	359 consecutive patients with community-acquired pneumonia.
Follow-up	A standardized evaluation, including specialized tests for Legionella species, and Chlamydia pneumoniae.

New and Emerging Etiologies for Community-Acquired
Pneumonia with Implications for Therapy:
A Prospective, Multicenter Study of 359 Cases.

(continued)

Results   The most common underlying illnesses were immuno-
             suppression (36.3%), chronic obstructive pulmonary dis-
             ease (32.4%), and malignancy (28.4%). The most frequent
             etiologic agents were Streptococcus pneumoniae
             (15.3%), and Hemophilus influenzae (10.9%). Surprisingly,
             Legionella species and C. pneumoniae were the third and
             fourth most frequent etiologies at 6.7% and 6.1%, respec-
             tively. Aerobic gram-negative pneumonias were relatively
             uncommon causes of pneumonia, despite the fact that
             empiric broad-spectrum combination antibiotic therapy
             is so often directed at this subgroup. In 32.9%, the etiolo-
             gy was undetermined. Antibiotic administration before
             admission was significantly associated with undetermined
             etiology (p=0.0003). There were no distinctive clinical fea-
             tures found to be diagnostic for any etiologic agent,
             although high fever occurred more frequently in
             Legionnaires' disease. Clinical manifestations for C. pneu-
             moniae were generally mild, although 38% of patients had
             mental status changes. Mortality was highest for
             Staphylococcus aureus (50%) and lowest for C. pneumo-
             niae (4.5%) and Mycoplasma pneumoniae (0%).

Conclusion   Specialized laboratory testing for C. pneumoniae and
             Legionella species should be more widely used rather
             than reserved for cases not responding to standard thera-
             py. Furthermore, realization that C. pneumoniae and
             Legionella species are common etiologies for communi-
             ty-acquired pneumonia should affect empiric antibiotic
             prescription.

Variations in Antimicrobial Use and Cost in More Than 2000 Patients with Community-Acquired Pneumonia

Title	Variations in antimicrobial use and cost in more than 2000 patients with community-acquired pneumonia.
Authors	Gilbert K, Gleason PP, Singer DE, et al.
Reference	Am J Med 1998;104:17–27.
Disease/ Pathogen	Pneumonia.
Purpose	To assess the patterns of antimicrobial use, costs of antimicrobial therapy, and medical outcomes by institution, in patients with community-acquired pneumonia.
Design	Prospective, multicenter, cohort study.
Patients	927 outpatients and 1328 inpatients enrolled in the pneumonia Patient Outcomes Research Team (PORT) multicenter, prospective cohort study.
Follow-up	Total antimicrobial costs were estimated by summing drug costs, using average wholesale price for oral agents, and institutional acquisition prices for parenteral agents, plus the costs associated with preparation and administration of parenteral therapy. Thirty-day outcome measures were mortality, subsequent hospitalization for outpatients, and hospital readmission for inpatients.

Results

Significant variation (p<0.05) in prescribing practices occurred for 17 of the 23 antimicrobial agents used in outpatients across five treatment sites, and for 18 of the 20 parenteral agents used in inpatients across four treatment sites. The median duration of antimicrobial therapy for treatment site ranged from 11 to 13 days for outpatients (p=0.01), and from 13 to 15 days for inpatients (p=0.49). The overall median cost of antimicrobial therapy was $12.90 for outpatients, and ranged from $10.80 to $58.90 among treatment sites (p<0.0001). The overall median cost of antimicrobial therapy was $228.70 for inpatients, and ranged from $183.70 to $315.60 among sites (p<0.0001). Mortality and hospital readmission for inpatients were not significantly different across sites after adjusting for baseline differences in patient demographic characteristics, comorbidity, and illness severity. Although subsequent hospitalization for outpatients differed by site, the rate was lowest for the site with the lowest antimicrobial costs.

Conclusion

Variations in antimicrobial prescribing practices by treatment site exist for outpatients and inpatients with community-acquired pneumonia. Although variation in antimicrobial prescribing practices across institutions results in significant differences in antimicrobial costs, patients treated at institutions with the lowest antimicrobial costs do not demonstrate worse medical outcomes.

A Prospective Study of the Impact of Community-Based Azithromycin Treatment of Trachoma on Carriage and Resistance of Streptococcus Pneumoniae

Title	A prospective study of the impact of community-based azithromycin treatment of trachoma on carriage and resistance of Streptococcus pneumoniae.
Authors	Leach AJ, Shelby-James TM, Mayo M, et al.
Reference	Clin Infect Dis 1997;24(3):356–362.
Disease/ Pathogen	Streptococcal pneumonia.
Purpose	To study the impact of community-based azithromycin treatment of trachoma on carriage and resistance of Streptococcus pneumonia.
Design	Prospective.
Patients	Children with trachoma and their houshold contacts.
Follow-up	2–3 weeks, 2 months, and 6 months after treatment.
Treatment/ prophylaxis regimen	Single-dose azithromycin was given to children with trachoma, and their household contacts who were children.

A Prospective Study of the Impact of Community-Based Azithromycin Treatment of Trachoma on Carriage and Resistance of Streptococcus Pneumoniae

(continued)

Results

For children with trachoma, rates of carriage of pneumococci immediately before treatment with azithromycin and 2–3 weeks, 2 months, and 6 months after treatment were 68%, 29%, 78%, and 87%, respectively. The proportion of carriage-positive children with azithromycin-resistant Streptococcus pneumoniae strains was 1 of 54 (1.9%) before treatment, and then six of 11 (54.5%), 10 of 29 (34.5%), and two of 34 (5.9%) at follow-up visits. The profile of pneumococcal serotypes changed after azithromycin treatment. Azithromycin-resistant strains (serotypes 10F, 23A, and 45) were isolated from one (1.3%) of 79 pretreatment swab specimens, from 16 (21.3%) of 75 swab specimens collected up to 2 months after treatment, and from two (6%) of 32 obtained 6 months after treatment. Mathematical modeling showed a more rapid appearance of azithromycin-resistant pneumococcal strains in previously colonized children than in previously noncolonized children.

Conclusion

The selective effect of azithromycin allowed the growth and transmission of pre-existing azithromycin-resistant strains. More research is needed to clarify the clinical relevance and implications of azithromycin use.

A Randomized, Controlled Trial of Filgrastim as an Adjunct to Antibiotics for Treatment of Hospitalized Patients with Community-Acquired Pneumonia

Title	A randomized, controlled trial of filgrastim as an adjunct to antibiotics for treatment of hospitalized patients with community-acquired pneumonia.
Authors	Nelson S, Belknap SM, Carlson RW, et al.
Reference	J Infect Dis 1998;178(4):1075–1080.
Disease/ Pathogen	Community-acquired pneumonia.
Purpose	To evaluate the effect of filgrastim as an adjunt to antibiotics for the treatment of hospitalized patients with community-acquired pneumonia.
Design	Randomized, placebo controlled, multicenter trial.
Patients	Hospitalized patients with community-acquired pneumonia.
Follow-up	Outcome measures included time to resolution of morbidity (TRM, a composite measure of temperature, respiratory rate, blood oxygenation, and chest radiograph), 28-day mortality, length of stay, and adverse events.
Treatment/ prophylaxis regimen	Filgrastim (300 micrograms/day up to 10 days) as an adjunct to antibiotics was conducted for these patients.

A Randomized, Controlled Trial of Filgrastim as an Adjunct to Antibiotics for Treatment of Hospitalized Patients with Community-Acquired Pneumonia

(continued)

Results	Filgrastim increased blood neutrophils three-fold, but TRM, mortality, and length of hospitalization were not affected. Treatment, however, accelerated radiologic improvement and appeared to reduce serious complications (e.g., empyema, adult respiratory distress syndrome, and disseminated intravascular coagulation).
Conclusion	Filgrastim administration was safe and well tolerated in these patients. Additional trials are needed to establish the value of this approach to treatment of infectious diseases.

1. Syndromes

s. Sepsis/ Immunoprophylaxis

Treatment of Gram-Negative Bacteremia and Septic Shock with HA-1A Human Monoclonal Antibody Against Endotoxin: A Randomized, Double Blind, Placebo Controlled Trial.

Title	Treatment of gram-negative bacteremia and septic shock with HA-1A human monoclonal antibody against endo-toxin: A randomized, double blind, placebo controlled trial.
Authors	Ziegler EJ, Fisher CJ Jr, Sprung CL, et al.
Reference	N Engl J Med 1991;324:429–436.
Disease/ Pathogen	Bacteremia.
Purpose	To evaluate the efficacy and safety of HA-1A.
Design	Randomized, double blind trial, placebo controlled.
Patients	Patients with sepsis and a presumed diagnosis of gram-negative infection.
Treatment/ prophylaxis regimen	Patients received either a single 100-mg intravenous dose of HA-1A (in 3.5 g of albumin) or placebo (3.5 g of albumin).
Additional therapy	Other interventions, including the administration of antibiotics and fluids, were not affected by the study protocol.

Treatment of Gram-Negative Bacteremia and Septic Shock with HA-1A Human Monoclonal Antibody Against Endotoxin: A Randomized, Double Blind, Placebo Controlled Trial

(continued)

Results
Of 543 patients with sepsis who were treated, 200 (37%) had gram-negative bacteremia as proved by blood culture. For the patients with gram-negative bacteremia followed to death or day 28, there were 45 deaths among the 92 recipients of placebo (49%) and 32 deaths among the 105 recipients of HA-1A (30%; p=0.014). For the patients with gram-negative bacteremia and shock at entry, there were 27 deaths among the 47 recipients of placebo (57%) and 18 deaths among the 54 recipients of HA-1A (33%; p=0.017). Analyses that stratified according to the severity of illness at entry showed improved survival with HA-1A treatment in both severely ill and less severely ill patients. Of the 196 patients with gram-negative bacteremia who were followed to hospital discharge or death, 45 of the 93 given placebo (48%) were discharged alive, as compared with 65 of the 103 treated with HA-1A (63%; p=0.038). No benefit of treatment with HA-1A was demonstrated in the 343 patients with sepsis who did not prove to have gram-negative bacteremia. For all 543 patients with sepsis who were treated, the mortality rate was 43% among the recipients of placebo and 39% among those given HA-1A (p=0.24). All patients tolerated HA-1A well, and no anti-HA-1A antibodies were detected.

Conclusion
HA-1A is safe and effective for the treatment of patients with sepsis and gram-negative bacteremia.

Immunoprophylaxis Against Klebsiella and Pseudomonas Aeruginosa Infections

Title	Immunoprophylaxis against Klebsiella and Pseudomonas aeruginosa infections.
Authors	Donta ST, Peduzzi P, Cross AS, et al.
Reference	J Infect Dis 1996;174(3):537–543.
Disease/ Pathogen	Klebsiella and Pseudomonas aeruginosa infections.
Purpose	To determine if passive immunization could decrease the incidence or severity of Klebsiella and Pseudomonas aeruginosa infections.
Design	Randomized, placebo controlled trial.
Patients	Patients with klebsiella and pseudomonas infection who were admitted to intensive care units of 16 Department of Veterans Affairs and Department of Defense hospitals.
Treatment/ prophylaxis regimen	Patients were randomized to receive either 100 mg/kg intravenous hyperimmune globulin (IVIG), derived from donors immunized with a 24-valent klebsiella capsular polysaccharide plus an 8-valent P. aeruginosa O-polysaccharide-toxin A conjugate vaccine, or an albumin placebo.

Results
and
Conclusion

The overall incidence and severity of vaccine-specific klebsiella plus pseudomonas infections were not significantly different between the groups receiving albumin and IVIG. There was some evidence that IVIG may decrease the incidence (2.7% albumin vs 1.2% IVIG) and severity (1% vs 0.3%) of vaccine-specific Klebsiella infections, but these reductions were not statistically significant. The trial was stopped because it was statistically unlikely that IVIG would be protective against pseudomonas infections at the dosage being used. Patients receiving IVIG had more adverse reactions (14.4% vs 9.2%).

Excess Mortality in Critically Ill Patients with Nosocomial Bloodstream Infections

Title	Excess mortality in critically ill patients with nosocomial bloodstream infections.
Authors	Smith RL, Meixler SM, Simberkoff MS.
Reference	Chest 1991;100(1):164–167.
Purpose	To determine the excess mortality attributable to hospital-acquired bloodstream infections.
Design	The study included primary bloodstream infections, defined by a positive blood culture at least three days after hospitalization, in the absence of any other apparent source of infection.
Results	The most frequent blood isolates included Staphylococcus aureus (39%), gram-negative rods (24%), and Candida albicans (15%). The spectrum of blood isolates suggested that most infections were related to intravascular catheters. In a control group of intensive care unit patients (n=384), the death rate predicted by Acute Physiology and Chronic Health Evaluation (APACHE II) was similar to the observed death rate (35.3% vs 37.8%). In a subgroup of control patients (n=34), chosen for APACHE II scores that matched the patients with bloodstream infections, predicted and observed death rates were also similar (53.1% vs 52.9%). For patients with bloodstream infection, however, observed mortality (82.4%) significantly exceeded the predicted value (54.1%, p=0.025).
Conclusion	The authors conclude that critically ill patients who develop nosocomial bloodstream infections are at greater risk of death than patients with comparable severity of illness without this complication. The difference between the observed and predicted death rates, 28%, represents the excess mortality associated with bloodstream infection in critically ill patients.

The Clinical Significance of Positive Blood Cultures in the 1990s: A Prospective, Comprehensive Evaluation of the Microbiology, Epidemiology, and Outcome of Bacteremia and Fungemia in Adults.

Title	The clinical significance of positive blood cultures in the 1990s: A prospective, comprehensive evaluation of the microbiology, epidemiology, and outcome of bacteremia and fungemia in adults.
Authors	Weinstein MP, Towns ML, Quartey SM, et al.
Reference	Clin Infect Dis 1997;24(4):584–602.
Disease/ Pathogen	Septicemia.
Purpose	To assess clincal significance of positive blood cultures, we reviewed 843 episodes of positive blood cultures.
Design	Prospective study.
Patients	707 patients with septicemia.

The Clinical Significance of Positive Blood Cultures in the 1990s: A Prospective, Comprehensive Evaluation of the Microbiology, Epidemiology, and Outcome of Bacteremia and Fungemia in Adults.

(continued)

Results

The five most common pathogens were Staphylococcus aureus, Escherichia coli, coagulase-negative staphylococci (CNS), Klebsiella pneumoniae, and Enterococcus species. Although CNS were isolated most often, only 12.4% were clinically significant. Half of all episodes were nosocomial, and a quarter had no recognized source. Leading identifiable sources included intravenous catheters, the respiratory and genitourinary tracts, and intra-abdominal foci. Septicemia-associated mortality was 17.5%. Patients who received appropriate antimicrobial therapy throughout the course of infection had the lowest mortality (13.3%). Multivariate analysis showed that age (relative risk [RR] 1.80), micro-organism (RR 2.27), source of infection (RR 2.86), predisposing factors (RR 1.98), blood pressure (RR 2.29), body temperature (RR 2.04), and therapy (RR 2.72) independently influenced outcome.

Conclusion

Bloodstream infections in the 1990s are notable for the increased importance of CNS as both contaminants and pathogens, the proportionate increase in fungi and decrease in annaerobes as pathogens, the emergence of Mycobacterium avium complex as an important cause of bacteriam in patients with advance human immunodeficiency virus infection, and the reduction in mortality associated with infection.

The Natural History of the Systemic Inflammatory Response Syndrome (SIRS): A Prospective Study.

Title	The natural history of the systemic inflammatory response syndrome (SIRS): A Prospective study.
Authors	Rangel-Frausto MS, Pittet D, Costigan M, et al.
Reference	JAMA 1995;273(2):117–123.
Disease/ Pathogen	Systemic inflammatory response syndrome (SIRS).
Purpose	Define the epidemiology of the four recently classified syndromes describing the biologic response to infection: Systemic inflammaroty response syndroms (SIRS), sepsis, severe sepsis, and septic shock.
Design	Prospective cohort study with a follow-up of 28 days, or until discharge if earlier.
Patients	Patients were included if they met at least two of the criteria for SIRS: Fever or hypothermia, tachycardia, tachypnea, or abnormal white blood cell count.

The Natural History of the Systemic Inflammatory Response Syndrome (SIRS): A Prospective Study.

(continued)

Results
During the study period, 3708 patients were admitted to the survey units, and 2527 (68%) met the criteria for SIRS. The incidence density rates for SIRS in the surgical, medical, and cardiovascular intensive care units were 857, 804, and 542 episodes per 1000 patient-days, respectively, and 671, 495, and 320 per 1000 patient-days for the medical, cardiothoracic, and general surgery wards, respectively. Among patients with SIRS, 649 (26%) developed sepsis, 467 (18%) developed severe sepsis, and 110 (4%) developed septic shock. The median interval from SIRS to sepsis was inversely correlated with the number of SIRS criteria (two, three, or all four) that the patients met. As the population of patients progressed from SIRS to septic shock, increasing proportions had adult respiratory distress syndrome, disseminated intravascular coagulation, acute renal failure, and shock. Positive blood cultures were found in 17% of patients with sepsis, in 25% with severe sepsis, and in 69% with septic shock. There were also stepwise increases in mortality rates in the hierachy from SIRS, sepsis, severe sepsis, and septic shock: 7%, 16%, 20%, and 46%, respectively. Of interest, we also observed equal numbers of patients who appeared to have sepsis, severe sepsis, and septic shock, but who had negative cultures. They had been prescribed empirical antibiotics for a median of 3 days. The cause of the systemic inflammatory response in these culture-negative populations is unknown, but they had similar morbidity and mortality rates as the respective culture-positive populations.

Conclusion
This prospective, epidemiologic study of SIRS and related conditions provides, to our knowledge, the first evidence of a clinical progression from SIRS to sepsis to severe sepsis and septic shock.

Incidence, Risk Factors, and Outcome of Severe Sepsis and Septic Shock in Adults

Title	Incidence, risk factors, and outcome of severe sepsis and septic shock in adults.
Authors	Brun-Buisson C, Doyon F, Carlet J, et al.
Reference	JAMA 1995;274(12):968–974.
Purpose	To examine the incidence, risk factors, and oucome of severe sepsis in intensive care unit (ICU) patients.
Design	Inception cohort study from a 2-month prospective survey of 11,828 consecutive admissions to 170 adult ICUs of public hospitals in France.
Patients	Patients meeting clinical criteria for severe sepsis were included and classified as having documented infection (i.e., documented severe sepsis, n=742), or a clinical diagnosis of infection without microbiological documentation (i.e., culture-negative severe sepsis, n=310).

Results   Clinically suspected sepsis and confirmed severe sepsis occurred in 9 (95% confidence interval [CI] 8.5-9.5) and 6.3 (95% CI 5.8-6.7) of 100 ICU admissions, respectively. The 28-day mortality was 56% (95% CI 52%-60%) in patients with severe sepsis, and 60% (95% CI 55%-66%) in those with culture-negative severe sepsis. Major determinants of both early (<3 days) and secondary deaths in the whole cohort were the Simplified Acute Physiology Score (SAPS) II and the number of acute organ systme failures. Other risk factors for early death included a low arterial blood pH (<7.33) (p<0.001) and shock (p=0.03), whereas secondary deaths were associated with the admission category (p<0.001), a rapidly or ultimately fatal underlying disease (p<0.001), a pre-existing liver (p=0.01) or cardiovascular (p=0.002) insufficiency, hypothermia (p=0.02), thrombocytopenia (p=0.01), and multiple sources of infection (p=0.02). In patients with documented sepsis, bacteremia was associated with early mortality (p=0.03).

Conclusion   Only three of four patients presenting with clinically suspected severe sepsis have documented infection. However, patients with clinically suspected sepsis, but without microbiological documentation, and patients with documented infection share common risk factors and are at similarly high risk of death. In addition to the severity of illness score, acute organ failures and the characteristics of underlying disease should be accounted for in stratification of patients and outcome analyses.

1. Syndromes

t. Sexually Transmitted Diseases

A Randomized, Controlled Trial of a Behavioral Intervention to Prevent Sexually Transmitted Disease among Minority Women

Title	A randomized, controlled trial of a behavioral intervention to prevent sexually transmitted disease among minority women.
Authors	Shain RN, Piper JM, Newton ER, et al.
Reference	N Engl J Med 1999;340:93–100.
Disease/ Pathogen	Sexually transmitted diseases.
Purpose	To determine subsequent chlamydial or gonorrheal infection, which was evaluated on an intention-to-treat basis, by logistic-regression analysis.
Design	Randomized, controlled trial.
Patients	Women with nonviral sexually transmitted diseases in a randomized trial of a sex- and culture-specific behavioral intervention.
Follow-up	12 months.
Treatment/ prophylaxis regimen	The intervention consisted of three small-group sessions of 3–4 hours, each designed to help women recognize personal susceptibility, commit to changing their behaviors, and acquire necessary skills.

A Randomized, Controlled Trial of a Behavioral Intervention to Prevent Sexually Transmitted Disease among Minority Women

(continued)

Results

A total of 424 Mexican-American and 193 African-American women were enrolled; 313 were assigned to the intervention group. and 304 to the control group. The rate of participation in the intervention was 90%. The rates of retention in the sample were 82%, and 89% at the 6- and 12-month visits, respectively. Rates of subsequent infection were significantly lower in the intervention group than in the control group during the first 6 months (11.3% vs 17.2%, p=0.05), during the second 6 months (9.1% vs 17.7%, p=0.008), and over the entire 12-month study period (16.8% vs 26.9%, p=0.004).

Conclusion

A risk-reduction intervention consisting of three small-group sessions significantly decreased the rates of chlamydial and gonorrheal infection among Mexican-American and African-American women at high risk for sexually transmitted disease.

Improving Office-Based Physicians' Prevention Practices for Sexually Transmitted Diseases

Title	Improving office-based physicians' prevention practices for sexually transmitted diseases.
Authors	Rabin DL, Boekeloo BO, Marx ES, et al.
Reference	Ann Intern Med 1994;121:513–519.
Disease/ Pathogen	Sexually transmitted diseases.
Purpose	To determine whether office-based interventions increase primary care physicians' risk assessment of and counseling practices for patients regarding sexually transmitted diseases and the human immunodeficiency virus (HIV).
Design	Randomized, controlled, clinical trial.
Patients	757 office-based primary care physicians (family or general practice, internal medicine, and obstetrics-gynecology) interviewed by telephone before and after the intervention.
Follow-up	The survey after the intervention was done an average of 9 months after the initial survey, and physicians were visited by simulated patient evaluators an average of 11 months after the initial survey.
Treatment/ prophylaxis regimen	Mailed educational materials alone or coupled with a simulated patient instructor office visit.

Results	89% of physicians who received both educational materials and a simulated patient instructor visit reported that they reviewed the educational materials, compared with 53% of those who only received the educational materials ($p \leq 0.001$). Physicians in the combined intervention group had higher self-reported and observed rates for several risk assessment questions and counseling recommendations than did physicians in the control group or the group that only received educational materials. 73% of physicians of the combined intervention group reported an increase in counseling patients about reducing risky sexual behavior compared with 53% of the group receiving only educational materials and 42% of the control group ($p \leq 0.001$).
Conclusion	Mailed educational materials combined with an office visit by a simulated patient instructor for role-play and feedback on clinical performance increased the frequency of office-based physicians' risk assessment and risk reduction counseling of patients for sexually transmitted diseases and HIV infection.

1. Syndromes

u. Sinusitis

Primary-Care-Based, Randomised, Placebo Controlled Trial of Antibiotic Treatment in Acute Maxillary Sinusitis

Title	Primary-care-based, randomised, placebo controlled trial of antibiotic treatment in acute maxillary sinusitis.
Authors	van Buchem FL, Knottnerus JA, Schrijnemaekers VJ, et al.
Reference	Lancet 1997;349:683–687.
Disease/ Pathogen	Acute maxillary sinusitis.
Purpose	To determine the efficacy of amoxycillin treatment for acute maxillary sinusitis patients presenting to general practice.
Design	Randomized, placebo controlled.
Patients	214 pateints with acute maxillary sinusitis determined radiographically.
Follow-up	Clinical course was assessed after 1 week and 2 weeks, and reported relapses and complications were recorded during the following year.
Treatment/ prophylaxis regimen	Pateints were randomly assigned treatment with amoxycillin (750 mg three times daily for 7 days; n=108) or placebo (n=106).

Results   After 2 weeks, symptoms had improved substantially or disappeared in 83% of patients in the study group, and 77% of patients taking placebo. Amoxycillin did not influence the clinical course of maxillary sinusitis, nor the frequency of relapses during the 1-year follow-up. Radiographs had no prognostic value, nor were they an effect modifier. Side-effects were recorded in 28% of patients given amoxycillin, and in 9% of those taking placebo (p<0.01). The occurrence of relapse was similar in both groups (21% vs 17%) during the follow-up year.

Conclusion   Antibiotic treatment did not improve the clinical course of acute maxillary sinusitis presenting to general practice. For these patients, an initial radiographic examination is not necessary, and initial management can be limited to symptomatic treatment. Whether antibiotics are necessary in more severe cases warrants further study.

Randomized, Controlled Trial of 3 Vs 10 Days of Trimethoprim/Sulfamethoxazole for Acute Maxillary Sinusitis

Title	Randomized, controlled trial of 3 vs 10 days of trimethoprim/sulfamethoxazole for acute maxillary sinusitis.
Authors	Williams JW Jr., Holleman DR Jr., Samsa GP, et al.
Reference	JAMA 1995;273(13):1015–1021.
Disease/ Pathogen	Acute maxillary sinusitis.
Purpose	To compare 14-day outcomes and relapse and recurrence rates among patients with acute maxillary sinusitis randomized to 3-day (3D) vs 10-day (10D) treatment with trimethoprim/sulfamethoxazole (TMP/SMX).
Design	Randomized, placebo controlled trial.
Patients	Consecutive patients with sinus symptoms and radiographic evidence of maxillary sinusitis (complete opacity, air-fluid level, or ≥6 mm of mucosal thickening). Patients were excluded for antibiotic use within the past week, TMP/SMX allergy, symptoms for more than 30 days, or previous sinus surgery.
Follow-up	Radiographs were scored at baseline and 14 days by radiologists masked to clinical symptoms and treatment assignment. The primary outcome was number of days to "cure" or "much improvement" in sinus symptoms. Patients who were clinical successes by day 14 were assessed for symptomatic relapse or recurrence at 30 and 60 days, respectively.

Randomized, Controlled Trial of 3 Vs 10 Days of Trimethoprim/Sulfamethoxazole for Acute Maxillary Sinusitis

(continued)

Treatment/ prophylaxis regimen	All subjects (n=80) received oxymetazoline nasal spray 0.05%, two sprays twice daily for 3 days. Subjects were randomly assigned to TMP/SMX double strength: One tablet twice daily for 10 days or one tablet twice daily for 3 days followed by 7 days of placebo. At 7 and 14 days, patients rated their overall sinus symptoms on a Likert scale.
Results	Groups were comparable at randomization: Male, 100%; black, 53%; median age, 48 years (interquartile range, 41–63 years); symptom duration, 10 days (interquartile range, 6–17 days); bilateral maxillary disease, 51%; and radiograph score, 4 (interquartile range, 2–4). Outcome assessment was completed in 95% of patients at day 14 (n=76). Medication side effects and use of nonstudy sinus medications were equal between groups. By 14 days, 77% of 3D subjects and 76% of 10D subjects rated their sinus symptoms as cured, or much improved (95% confidence interval for difference [CI] -15%–17%). Median days to cure/much improvement were 5 and 4.5 for the 3D and 10D groups, respectively. Distributions of time to cure were not different (p=0.34). Radiograph scores improved in both groups compared with baseline (2 points; p<0.001), but improvement did not differ between groups (p=0.31). 8% of 3D subjects, and 13% of 10D subjects missed work due to sinus symptoms. Of the 52 patients who were clinical successes at 14 days and completed follow-up, three of 27 (11%) 3D subjects and one of 25 (4%) 10D subjects relapsed symptomatically by day 30; one of 27 (4%) 3D subjects and one of 25 (4%) 10D subjects suffered symptomatic recurrence between days 30 and 60 (p=0.45 for the relapse and recurrence rates combined).
Conclusion	At the 2-week follow-up, clinical symptoms and radiograph scores improved equally following 3 or 10 days of TMP/SMX plus oxymetazoline nasal spray. Symptomatic relapse and recurrence were similar between groups. Three days of antibiotics were as effective as 10 days and, because of the high disease prevalence, hold the potential for substantial cost savings.

1. Syndromes

v. Surgical Wound Infections

The Timing of Prophylactic Administration of Antibiotics and the Risk of Surgical-Wound Infection

Title	The timing of prophylactic administration of antibiotics and the risk of surgical-wound infection.
Authors	Classen DC, Evans RS, Pestotnik SL, et al.
Reference	N Engl J Med 1992;326(5):281–286.
Disease/ Pathogen	Surgical-wound infection.
Purpose	To determine how the timing of antibiotic administration affects the risk of surgical-wound infection in actual clinical practice.
Design	Randomized trial.
Patients	2847 patients undergoing elective clean or "clean-contaminated" surgical procedures at a large community hospital.
Treatment/ prophylaxis regimen	The administration of antibiotics 2–24 hours before the surgical incision was defined as early; that during the 2 hours before the incision, as pre-operative; that during the 3 hours after the incision, as peri-operative; and that >3, but <24 hours after the incision, as postoperative.

Results   Of the 1708 patients who received the prophylactic antibiotics pre-operatively, 10 (0.6%) subsequently had surgical-wound infections. Of the 282 patients who received the antibiotics peri-operatively, four (1.4%) had such infections (p=0.12; relative risk [RR] as compared with the preoperatively treated group, 2.4; 95% confidence interval [CI] 0.9-7.9). Of 488 patients who received the antibiotics postoperatively, 16 (3.3%) had wound infections (p<0.0001; RR 5.8; 95% CI 2.6-12.3). Finally, of 369 patients who had antibiotics administered early, 14 (3.8%) had wound infections (p<0.0001; RR 6.7; 95% CI 2.9-14.7). Stepwise logistic-regression analysis confirmed that the administration of antibiotics in the pre-operative period was associated with the lowest risk of surgical-wound infection.

Conclusion   The authors conclude that in surgical practice there is considerable variation in the timing of prophylactic administration of antibiotics and that administration in the two hours before surgery reduces the risk of wound infection.

1. Syndromes
w. Urethritis

Azithromycin for Empirical Treatment of the Nongonococcal Urethritis Syndrome in Men: A Randomized, Double Blind Study.

Title	Azithromycin for empirical treatment of the nongonococcal urethritis syndrome in men: A randomized, double blind study.
Authors	Stamm WE, Hicks CB, Martin DH, et al.
Reference	JAMA 1995;274:545–549.
Disease/ Pathogen	Nongonococcal urethritis.
Purpose	To evaluate the use of single-dose azithromycin for empirical treatment of nongonococcal urethritis.
Design	Randomized, double blind, multicenter trial comparing azithromycin vs doxycycline therapy, with a 2:1 randomization ratio.
Patients	A total of 452 men aged 18 years or older with symptomatic nongonococcal urethritis of less than 14 days' duration.
Follow-up	Clinical resolution of symptoms and signs of nongonococcal urethritis, microbiological cure of C. trachomatis and Ureaplasma urealyticum, and occurrence of adverse experiences.
Treatment/ prophylaxis regimen	Patients were treated with either 1 g of azithromycin as a single oral dose or 100 mg of doxycycline taken orally twice daily for 7 days.

(continued)

Results
: Of the 452 patients enrolled, 248 in the azithromycin-treated group and 123 in the doxycycline-treated group were evaluable for clinical response. The two treatment groups were comparable in terms of age, weight, ethnic distribution, sexual preference, sexual activity, and history of prior nongonococcal urethritis or gonorrhea. Sixteen percent of the azithromycin group and 24% of the doxycycline group were culture positive for C. trachomatis before therapy, while 38% and 28%, respectively, were culture positive for U. urealyticum. The cumulative clinical cure rate was 81% (95% confidence interval [CI] 75%-85%) in the azithromycin-treated group and 77% (95% CI 69%-84%) in the doxycycline-treated group. Clinical cure rates in the two groups were also comparable when patients were stratified by presence or absence of infection with C. trachomatis or U. urealyticum prior to therapy. Among those infected with C. trachomatis, overall microbiological cure rates were 83% (95% CI 65%-94%) for azithromycin-treated patients (n=30) and 90% (95% CI 68%-98%) for doxycycline-treated patients (n=21). Among those infected with U. urealyticum, overall microbiological cure rates were 45% (95% CI 34%-57%) for azithromycin-treated patients (n=75) and 47% (95% CI, 30%-65%) for doxycycline-treated patients (n=32). Adverse reactions were generally mild to moderate and occurred in 23% of the azithromycin-treated group and 29% of the doxycycline-treated group.

Conclusion
: For empirical treatment of the acute nongonococcal urethritis syndrome in men, a single oral dose of azithromycin was as effective as a standard 7-day course of doxycycline in achieving clinical cure. Further, clinical cure rates were comparable with either regimen, regardless of the presence or absence of chlamydia or ureaplasma infection.

1. Syndromes

x. Urinary Tract Infection

Title	Prevalence of asymptomatic bacteriuria and associated host factors in women with diabetes mellitus.
Authors	Zhanel GG, Nicolle LE, Harding GK.
Reference	Clin Infect Dis 1995;21(2):316–322.
Disease/ Pathogen	Asymptomatic bacteruria.
Purpose	To determine the prevalence of significant asymptomatic bacteriuria in adult women with diabetes mellitus attending endocrinology clinics at two tertiary-care university-affiliated teaching hospitals.
Design	Prospective study.
Patients	85 bacteriuric and 987 nonbacteriuric women.
Results	The overall prevalence of bacteriuria was 7.9% (85 cases per 1072 women). Absolute urinary leukocyte (white blood cell) counts were $\geq 10/mm^3$ in 77.6% (66) of the 85 bacteriuric women vs 23.7% (234) of the 987 nonbacteriuric women (p<0.001). Bacteriuric women were significantly more likely than nonbacteriuric women to have non-insulin-dependent diabetes mellitus, longer duration of diabetes, neuropathy, and heart disease. Aboriginals had bacteriuria at a significantly higher prevalence rate than that among nonaboriginals (19.7% [15 of 76] vs 7% [70 of 996], respectively; p<0.0001), were more likely to have occult upper urinary tract infection (antibody-coated bacteria positivity: 53% [8 of 15] vs 20% [10 of 50], respectively; p=0.016), and had significantly lower urinary leukocyte counts, whether they were bacteriuric or not (p<0.05).

| Conclusion | Multivariate analysis identified duration of diabetes and aboriginal origin as independent risk factors for the presence of bacteriuria. |

Does Eradicating Bacteriuria Affect the Severity of Chronic Urinary Incontinence in Nursing Home Residents?

Title	Does eradicating bacteriuria affect the severity of chronic urinary incontinence in nursing home residents?
Authors	Ouslander JG, Schapira M, Schnelle JF, et al.
Reference	Ann Intern Med 1995;122:749–754.
Disease/ Pathogen	Urinary tract infection.
Purpose	To determine the effects of eradicating otherwise asymptomatic bacteriuria on the severity of chronic urinary incontinence among nursing home residents.
Design	Randomized, controlled, multicenter.
Patients	Nursing home residents with chronic urinary incontinence.
Follow-up	3 days.
Treatment/ prophylaxis regimen	The immediate treatment group received antimicrobial therapy for 7 days; after outcome measures had been repeated, the delayed treatment group was treated.

Results   191 residents were enrolled, and 176 completed the study. Bacteriuria was eradicated by antimicrobial therapy in 71 residents (40%), and 17 residents (10%) had bacteriuria before and after therapy. The percentage of hourly checks at which the residents were found wet, and other measures of incontinence severity remained essentially the same after bacteriuria was eradicated. In the nonbacteriuric group, the percentage of checks that were wet increased from 29% (95% confidence interval [CI] 26%-32%) at baseline to 30% (CI 27%-34%) on repeated measurement. In the bacteriuric groups, the percentage increased from 34% (CI 30%-38%) before treatment to 35% (CI 31%-39%) after bacteriuria was eradicated. The presence of pyuria did not affect the results.

Conclusion   Eradicating bacteriuria has no short-term effects on the severity of chronic urinary incontinence among nursing home residents. Our data support the practice of not treating asymptomatic bacteriuria in this population and validate the recommendations in the Health Care Financing Administration's Resident Assessment Protocol for urinary incontinence.

Does Asymptomatic Bacteriuria Predict Mortality and Does Antimicrobial Treatment Reduce Mortality in Elderly Ambulatory Women?

Title	Does asymptomatic bacteriuria predict mortality and does antimicrobial treatment reduce mortality in elderly ambulatory women?
Authors	Abrutyn E, Mossey J, Berlin JA, et al.
Reference	Ann Intern Med 1994;120:827–833.
Disease/ Pathogen	Urinary tract infection.
Purpose	To determine whether asymptomatic bacteriuria in elderly ambulatory women is a marker of increased mortality and, if so, whether it is because of an association with other determinants of mortality or because asymptomatic bacteriuria is itself an independent cause; the removal of which might improve longevity.
Design	A cohort study and a controlled clinical trial of the effect of antimicrobial treatment.
Patients	Women without urinary tract catheters (observational study, n=1491), (clinical trial, n=358).
Follow-up	Urine cultures every 6 months (the same organism at 10(5) colony-forming units or more per mL on two midstream urine specimens defined asymptomatic bacteriuria), comorbidity, and mortality.

Does Asymptomatic Bacteriuria Predict Mortality and Does Antimicrobial Treatment Reduce Mortality in Elderly Ambulatory Women?

(continued)

Treatment/ prophylaxis regimen	Culture-positive patients were assigned to antimicrobial treatment or placebo. Single-dose therapy was given with trimethoprim, 200 mg, or norfloxacin, 400 mg, depending on the susceptibility of the organism. The same drugs (trimethoprim, 100 mg twice daily, and norfloxacin, 400 mg twice daily) were used for 14 days of therapy in patients failing single-dose therapy.
Results	In the observational study, infected residents (n=318) were older, and sicker, and had higher mortality (18.7 per 100,000 resident-days) than uninfected residents (n=1173; 10.1 per 100,000 resident-days). However, in a multivariate Cox analysis, infection was not related to mortality (relative risk 1.1; p>0.2), whereas age at entry and self-rated health (score 1 [excellent] to 4 [bad or poor]) were strong predictors. In the clinical trial, mortality in 166 treated residents (13.8 per 100,000 resident-days) was comparable to that of 192 untreated residents (15.1 per 100,000 resident-days); the relative rate was 0.92 (95% confidence interval 0.57–1.47). The cure rates among treated and untreated residents were 82.9% and 15.6%, respectively.
Conclusion	Urinary tract infection was not an independent risk factor for mortality, and its treatment did not lower the mortality rate. Screening and treatment of asymptomatic bacteriuria in ambulatory elderly women to decrease mortality do not appear warranted.

Title	Diagnosis of urinary tract infection in children: Fresh urine microscopy or culture?
Authors	Vickers D, Ahmad T, Coulthard MG.
Reference	Lancet 1991;338:767–770.
Disease/ Pathogen	Urinary tract infection (UTI).
Purpose	To compare diagnosis of a UTI in children using fresh urine microscopy or culture.
Design	Fresh unspun and unstained urine specimens were examined by microscopy at a magnification of x 400 in a mirrored counting chamber by a clinician, and sent for culture in a microbiology laboratory; 200 samples were also plated onto dip-slides.
Patients	342 children with previous UTI or symptoms compatible with an UTI.
Follow-up	When microscopy and culture results were discrepant, further urine samples were collected until a diagnosis of UTI (24) or sterile urine (318) could be confirmed.

Treatment/ prophylaxis regimen	Initial microscopy correctly identified 23 of 24 UTIs and 286 of 318 sterile urines; 1 false-positive result was caused by vaginal contamination with lactobacilli. 32 specimens (9%) gave an equivocal result on microscopy; the one other true-positive result was identified correctly on microscopy of the next urine specimen obtained. Culture of the initial urines correctly identified all 24 UTIs, but only 82% of the negative samples. Of the samples from uninfected children, 35 (11%) showed a mixed growth which was sterile on repeat sampling, and 21 (6.6%) initially grew a false-positive pure growth of more than 10(5) colony-forming units/ml of one organism. True UTIs were associated with bacterial counts above 10(7)/ml.
Conclusion	Microscopy by a clinician represents a cheaper, quicker, and more reliable screening test for UTI in children than does routine culture in a microbiology laboratory.

Postcoital Antimicrobial Prophylaxis for Recurrent Urinary Tract Infection: A Randomized, Double Blind, Placebo Controlled Trial.

Title	Postcoital antimicrobial prophylaxis for recurrent urinary tract infection: A randomized, double blind, placebo controlled trial.
Authors	Stapleton A, Latham RH, Johnson C, et al.
Reference	JAMA 1990;264:703–706.
Disease/ Pathogen	Urinary tract infection.
Purpose	To determine the efficacy of postcoital antibiotic prophylaxis in healthy young women prone to recurrent urinary tract infections.
Design	Randomized, double blind, placebo controlled study.
Patients	16 women patients.
Follow-up	6 months of observation.
Treatment/ prophylaxis regimen	Sixteen patients were randomized to receive postcoital administration of a combination product of trimethoprim and sulfamethoxazole, while 11 received postcoital placebo.

Postcoital Antimicrobial Prophylaxis for Recurrent Urinary Tract Infection: A Randomized, Double Blind, Placebo Controlled Trial.

(continued)

Results In over 6 months of observation, postcoital administration of trimethoprim-sulfamethoxazole was highly effective in preventing recurrent urinary tract infections. Nine of 11 patients who took the placebo developed urinary tract infections (infection rate, 3.6 per patient-year), compared with only two of 16 patients who received postcoital trimethoprim-sulfamethoxazole (infection rate, 0.3 per patient-year). Postcoital administration of trimethoprim-sulfamethoxazole was effective in patients with both low (two or fewer times per week) and high (three or more times per week) intercourse frequencies. Side effects were few and compliance was excellent.

Conclusion The authors conclude that postcoital trimethoprim-sulfamethoxazole is a safe, effective, and inexpensive approach to management of recurrent urinary tract infections in young women.

A Randomized Trial of Short-Course Ciprofloxacin, Ofloxacin, or Trimethoprim/Sulfamethoxazole for the Treatment of Acute Urinary Tract Infection in Women

Title	A randomized trial of short-course ciprofloxacin, ofloxacin, or trimethoprim/sulfamethoxazole for the treatment of acute urinary tract infection in women.
Authors	McCarty JM, Richard G, Huck W, et al.
Reference	Am J Med 1999;106:292–299.
Disease/ Pathogen	Urinary tract infection.
Purpose	This study reports the results of short-course ciprofloxacin, ofloxacin, and trimethoprim/sulfamethoxazole therapy for bladder infections in otherwise healthy women.
Design	Randomized, double blind study of the efficacy and safety of a 3-day course of oral ciprofloxacin, ofloxacin, or trimethoprim/sulfamethoxazole in women with accute, uncomplicated, symptomatic lower urinary tract infection.
Patients	A total of 866 patients with acute, uncomplicated, symptomatic lower urinary tract infection were enrolled; of whom 688 (79%) were evaluated for the efficacy of treatment (229 treated with ciprofloxacin, 228 treated with trimethoprim/sulfamethoxazole, and 231 treated with ofloxacin). The most frequent reason for exclusion was the failure to identify a pretreatment pathogen.
Follow-up	Follow-up at 4–6 weeks.

A Randomized Trial of Short-Course Ciprofloxacin, Ofloxacin, or Trimethoprim/Sulfamethoxazole for the Treatment of Acute Urinary Tract Infection in Women

(continued)

Treatment/ prophylaxis regimen	A 3-day course of oral ciprofloxacin 100 mg twice daily, ofloxacin 200 mg twice daily, or trimethoprim/sulfamethoxazole 160/800 mg twice daily.
Results	The most commonly isolated pathogen was Escherichia coli (81%). Eradication of the pretreatment pathogen at the end of therapy occurred in 94% of ciprofloxacin, 93% of trimethoprim/sulfamethoxazole, and 97% of ofloxacin-treated patients. At follow-up evaluation at 4-6 weeks, recurrence rates (relapse or reinfection) were 11% in the ciprofloxacin, 16% in the trimethoprim/sulfamethoxazole, and 13% in the ofloxacin treatment group. Clinical success at the end of therapy was 93% in the ciprofloxacin, 95% in the trimethoprim/sulfamethoxazole, and 96% in the ofloxacin treatment groups. The frequency of all adverse events was 31% for ciprofloxacin, 41% for trimethoprim/sulfamethoxazole, and 39% for ofloxacin-treated patients (p=0.03). Premature discontinuation of study drug due to an adverse event was more common in trimethoprim/sulfamethoxazole-treated patients (n=9) compared with those given ciprofloxacin (n=2) or ofloxacin (n=1; p=0.02).
Conclusion	Ciprofloxacin, ofloxacin, and trimethoprim/sulfamethoxazole had similar efficacy when given for 3 days to treat acute, symptomatic, uncomplicated lower urinary tract infection in women.

*Prophylaxis of Urinary Tract Infection in Persons with
Recent Spinal Cord Injury: A Prospective, Randomized,
Double Blind, Placebo Controlled Study
of Trimethoprim-Sulfamethoxazole.*

Title	Prophylaxis of urinary tract infection in persons with recent spinal cord injury: A prospective, randomized, double blind, placebo controlled study of trimethoprim-sulfamethoxazole.
Authors	Gribble MJ, Puterman ML.
Reference	Am J Med 1993;95(2):141–152.
Disease/ Pathogen	Urinary tract infection.
Purpose	To determine the efficacy of trimethoprim-sulfamethoxazole (TMP-SMX) for prophylaxis of urinary tract infection in persons with recent spinal cord injury, during the first 4 months of intermittent catheterization.
Design	Randomized, double blind, placebo controlled trial.
Patients	129 adults (112 men, 17 women) with recent acute spinal cord injury.
Follow-up	16 weeks. Clinical observations, urine cultures, and cultures of rectal and urethral swabs were made weekly. Subjects who developed breakthrough bacteriuria received conventional antimicrobial therapy and prophylaxis was continued.

Prophylaxis of Urinary Tract Infection in Persons with Recent Spinal Cord Injury: A Prospective, Randomized, Double Blind, Placebo Controlled Study of Trimethoprim-Sulfamethoxazole.

(continued)

Treatment/ prophylaxis regimen	Low-dose TMP-SMX (TMP 40 mg, SMX 200 mg) or placebo was given once daily.
Results	66 TMP-SMX recipients (57 men, 9 women) and 60 placebo recipients (52 men, 8 women) were evaluable for efficacy. Among male subjects, bacteriuria was present during 50% or more of study weeks in 30% of TMP-SMX recipients and in 56% of placebo recipients (p=0.003). The interval to the onset of bacteriuria was prolonged in TMP-SMX recipients (p<0.0001). TMP-SMX recipients without bacteriuria in any given week had a lower probability of having bacteriuria the subsequent week (0.26) than did placebo recipients (0.49) (p<0.0001). At least one episode of definite symptomatic bacteriuria (bacteriuria and fever and at least 1 classical manifestation of urinary infection) occurred in four of 57 TMP-SMX-treated men and in 18 of 52 placebo-treated men (p<0.0003). We observed similar trends in women, but differences did not reach statistical significance, perhaps because the number of females was small. Adverse events suspected to be due to medications were frequent in this population of patients with recent severe injuries and led to discontinuation of the study in 10% of the TMP-SMX group and 8% of the placebo group. Adverse events included neutropenia (TMP-SMX: Two; placebo: Three), pseudomembranous colitis (TMP-SMX: One), severe skin rash (TMP-SMX: Two; placebo: One), and drug fever (TMP-SMX: One). The proportion of all episodes of bacteriuria that were due to TMP-SMX-resistant organisms was unexpectedly high in the placebo group (51%), and increased progressively according to year of enrollment in the study. By year three, all subjects in the placebo group had at least one episode of TMP-SMX-resistant bacteriuria. Gram-negative enteric bacilli resistant to TMP-SMX were recovered from rectal swabs (TMP-SMX 49%, placebo 42%) and urethral swabs (TMP-SMX 33%, placebo 26%) in similar proportions of subjects in the two study groups.

***Prophylaxis of Urinary Tract Infection in Persons with
Recent Spinal Cord Injury: A Prospective, Randomized,
Double Blind, Placebo Controlled Study
of Trimethoprim-Sulfamethoxazole.***

(continued)

Conclusion   Prophylaxis with TMP-SMX significantly reduces bacteriuria and symptomatic urinary tract infection in persons
with recent acute spinal cord injury during bladder
retraining using intermittent catheterization. However,
adverse reactions attributable to TMP-SMX are common
in this population. Colonization and breakthrough bacteriuria with TMP-SMX-resistant organisms are frequent
and may seriously limit the usefulness of this strategy, particularly in an institutional setting.

Title	Randomized, comparative trial and cost analysis of 3-day antimicrobial regimens for treatment of acute cystitis in women.
Authors	Hooton TM, Winter C, Tiu F, et al.
Reference	JAMA 1995;273:41–45.
Disease/ Pathogen	Cystitis.
Purpose	To determine the efficacy, safety, and costs associated with four different 3-day regimens for the treatment of acute uncomplicated cystitis in women.
Design	A prospective, randomized trial with a cost analysis.
Patients	Women with acute cystitis attending a student health center.
Treatment/ prophylaxis regimen	Treatment with 3-day oral regimens of trimethoprim-sulfamethoxazole, 160 mg/800 mg twice daily, macrocrystalline nitrofurantoin, 100 mg four times daily, cefadroxil, 500 mg twice daily, or amoxicillin, 500 mg three times daily.

Randomized, Comparative Trial and Cost Analysis of 3-Day Antimicrobial Regimens for Treatment of Acute Cystitis in Women

(continued)

Results

6 weeks after treatment, 32 (82%) of 39 women treated with trimethoprim-sulfamethoxazole were cured, compared with 22 (61%) of 36 treated with nitrofurantoin (p=0.04 vs trimethoprim-sulfamethoxazole), 21 (66%) of 32 treated with cefadroxil (p=0.11 vs trimethoprim-sulfamethoxazole), and 28 (67%) of 42 treated with amoxicillin (p=0.11 vs trimethoprim-sulfamethoxazole). Persistence of significant bacteriuria was less common with trimethoprim-sulfamethoxazole (3%) and cefadroxil (0%), compared with nitrofurantoin (16%; p=0.05 vs trimethoprim-sulfamethoxazole) and amoxicillin (14%; p=0.11 vs trimethoprim-sulfamethoxazole). Persistence of bacteriuria was associated with amoxicillin-resistant strains in the amoxicillin group, but nitrofurantoin-susceptible strains in the nitrofurantoin group. Trimethoprim-sulfamethoxazole was more successful in eradicating Escherichia coli from rectal cultures soon after therapy and from urethral and vaginal cultures at all follow-up visits compared with the other treatment regimens. Adverse effects were reported by 16 (35%) of 46 patients receiving trimethoprim-sulfamethoxazole, 18 (43%) of 42 receiving nitrofurantoin, 12 (30%) of 40 receiving cefadroxil, and 13 (25%) of 52 receiving amoxicillin. The mean costs per patient were less with trimethoprim-sulfamethoxazole ($114) and amoxicillin ($131) compared with nitrofurantoin ($155) and cefadroxil ($155).

Conclusion

A 3-day regimen of trimethoprim-sulfamethoxazole is more effective and less expensive than 3-day regimens of nitrofurantoin, cefadroxil, or amoxicillin for treatment of uncomplicated cystitis in women. The increased efficacy of trimethoprim-sulfamethoxazole is likely related to its antimicrobial effects against E. coli in the rectum, urethra, and vagina.

2. Pathogens

a. Aspergillosis

Title	An European Organisation for Research and Treatment of Cancer (EORTC) international, multicenter, randomized trial (EORTC No. 19,923) comparing two dosages of liposomal amphotericin B for treatment of invasive aspergillosis.
Authors	Ellis M, Spence D, de Pauw B, et al.
Reference	Clin Infect Dis 1998;27(6):1406–1412.
Disease/ Pathogen	Aspergillosis.
Purpose	To compare the clinical efficacy of two dosages of liposomal amphotericin B (L-AmB) for IA in neutropenic patients with cancer or those undergoing bone marrow transplantation.
Design	Prospective randomized clinical trial.
Patients	Eighty-seven patients with invasive aspergillosis (IA).
Follow-up	Six months.
Treatment/ prophylaxis regimen	41 patients received 1 mg/(kg.d) (L-AmB-1) and of 46 received 4 mg/(kg.d) (L-AmB-4).

An EORTC International, Multicenter, Randomized Trial (EORTC No. 19,923) Comparing Two Dosages of Liposomal Amphotericin B for Treatment of Invasive Aspergillosis

(continued)

Results	Clinical responses were documented for 26 (64%) of 41 patients receiving 1 mg/(kg.d) (L-AmB-1) and 22 (48%) of 46 receiving 4 mg/(kg.d) (L-AmB-4). Radiologic response rates were similar: 24 (58%) of the L-AmB-1 recipients and 24 (52%) of the L-AmB-4 recipients. The 6-month survival rates were 43% (L-AmB-1) and 37% (L-AmB-4). These differences were not significant. The numbers of deaths directly due to IA at 6 months were similar: Nine (22%) of 41 L-AmB-1 recipients and nine (20%) of 46 L-AmB-4 recipients. No other variable independently influenced survival, apart from central nervous system IA.
Conclusion	L-AmB is effective in treating approximately 50%–60% of patients who have IA. A 1-mg/(kg.d) dosage is as effective as a 4-mg/(kg.d) dosage, and no advantages to use of the higher, more expensive, dosage has been observed.

Amphotericin B Colloidal Dispersion Vs Amphotericin B as Therapy for Invasive Aspergillosis

Title	Amphotericin B colloidal dispersion vs amphotericin B as therapy for invasive aspergillosis.
Authors	White MH, Anaissie EJ, Kusne S, et al.
Reference	Clin Infect Dis 1997;24(4):635–642.
Disease/ Pathogen	Aspergillosis.
Purpose	To compare the safety and efficacy of amphotericin B colloidal dispersion (ABCD) with amphotericin B for the treatment of invasive aspergillosis.
Design	Patients with proven or probable aspergillosis who were treated in clinical trials with ABCD were compared retrospectively with patients with aspergillosis who were treated with amphotericin B at six cancer or transplant centers from January 1990 to June 1994.
Patients	82 patients with proven or probable aspergillosis were treated with ABCD and 261 were treated with amphotericin B.
Treatment/ prophylaxis regimen	Patients received either ABCD or amphotericin B.

Amphotericin B Colloidal Dispersion Vs Amphotericin B as Therapy for Invasive Aspergillosis

(continued)

Results
: The groups were balanced in terms of underlying disease; ABCD recipients were younger and more likely to have pre-existing renal insufficiency than were amphotericin B recipients (40.7% vs 8.7%, respectively), and amphotericin B recipients were more likely to be neutropenic at baseline than were ABCD recipients (42.5% vs 15.9%, respectively). Response rates (48.8%) and survival rates (50%) among ABCD-treated patients were higher than those (23.4% and 28.4%, respectively) among amphotericin B-treated patients (p<0.001 for both comparisons). Renal dysfunction developed less frequently in ABCD recipients than in amphotericin B recipients (8.2% vs 43.1%, respectively; p<0.001). Multivariate analysis revealed that treatment group was the best predictor of response, mortality, and nephrotoxicity (ABCD: relative risk [RR]=3, p=0.002; RR=0.35, p<0.001; and RR=0.13, p=0.001, respectively).

Conclusion
: This retrospective study suggests that in the treatment of aspergillosis, ABCD causes fewer nephrotoxic effects than amphotericin B and the efficacy of ABCD is at least comparable with that of amphotericin B.

2. Pathogens

b. Atypical Mycobacterial Infections

Clarithromycin Resistance and Susceptibility Patterns of Mycobacterium Avium Strains Isolated During Prophylaxis for Disseminated Infection in Patients with AIDS

Title	Clarithromycin resistance and susceptibility patterns of Mycobacterium avium strains isolated during prophylaxis for disseminated infection in patients with AIDS.
Authors	Craft JC, Notario GF, Grosset JH, et al.
Reference	Clin Infect Dis 1998;27(4):807–812.
Disease/ Pathogen	Mycobacterium avium complex (MAC).
Purpose	To evaluate the efficacy of clarithromycin in the prevention of disseminated Mycobacterium avium complex (MAC) infection in patients with AIDS; special attention was given to the development of clarithromycin resistance.
Design	Randomized, placebo controlled trial.
Follow-up	The median time to document MAC bacteremia was 199 days for placebo-treated patients, 217 days for clarithromycin-treated patients infected with clarithromycin-susceptible MAC, and 385 days for clarithromycin-treated patients infected with clarithromycin-resistant MAC.
Results	Most of the patients with clarithromycin-resistant isolates (91%) had a baseline CD4 T-cell count of <20/microL, while these low counts occurred in only 25% of patients having clarithromycin-susceptible breakthrough isolates.

***Clarithromycin Resistance and Susceptibility Patterns of
Mycobacterium Avium Strains Isolated During Prophylaxis
for Disseminated Infection in Patients with AIDS***

(continued)

Conclusion   The emergence of clarithromycin resistance did not affect
the total period of survival. Resistance to clarithromycin
in breakthrough MAC isolates emerges most likely when
the patient is extremely immunodeficient at the time of
initiation of the preventative therapy.

Initial (6-Month) Results of Three-Times-Weekly Azithromycin in Treatment Regimens for Mycobacterium Avium Complex Lung Disease in Human Immunodeficiency Virus-Negative Patients

Title	Initial (6-month) results of three-times-weekly azithromycin in treatment regimens for Mycobacterium avium complex lung disease in human immunodeficiency virus-negative patients.
Authors	Griffith DE, Brown BA, Murphy DT, et al.
Reference	J Infect Dis 1998;178(1):121–126.
Disease/ Pathogen	Mycobacterium avium complex (MAC).
Purpose	To evaluate the effects of intermittent azithromycin (600 mg), usually given Monday, Wednesday, and Friday (TIW) for MAC lung disease in human immunodeficiency virus-negative patients.
Design	Two consecutive, open, prospective trials.
Patients	Patients with MAC who were human immunodeficiency virus-negative patients.
Treatment/ prophylaxis regimen	Regimen A consisted of TIW azithromycin and daily ethambutol (15 mg/kg/day), daily rifabutin (300 mg/day), and initial twice weekly (BIW) streptomycin. Regimen B consisted of TIW azithromycin, TIW ethambutol (25 mg/kg/dose), TIW rifabutin (600 mg/dose), and initial twice weekly streptomycin.

Initial (6-Month) Results of Three-Times-Weekly Azithromycin in Treatment Regimens for Mycobacterium Avium Complex Lung Disease in Human Immunodeficiency Virus-Negative Patients

(continued)

Results	Of 19 patients enrolled in regimen A who completed at least 6 months of therapy, 14 (74%) had sputum samples become culture-negative. Of 39 patients enrolled in regimen B who completed at least 6 months of therapy, 24 (62%) had sputum conversion. These sputum conversion rates are comparable to previous rates at 6 months in patients receiving daily clarithromycin- or azithromycin-containing regimens. No resistance to azithromycin emerged with either regimen.
Conclusion	This is the first study to demonstrate the efficacy of intermittent administration of medication for MAC lung disease.

2. Pathogens

c. Blastomycosis

Treatment of Blastomycosis with Higher Doses of Fluconazole

Title	Treatment of blastomycosis with higher doses of fluconazole.
Authors	Pappas PG, Bradsher RW, Kauffman CA, et al.
Reference	Clin Infect Dis 1997;25(2):200–205.
Disease/ Pathogen	Blastomycosis.
Purpose	To determine the efficacy and safety of two different daily doses of fluconazole (400 and 800 mg) in the treatment of non-life-threatening blastomycosis.
Design	Randomized, multicenter, open label study.
Patients	39 patients with blastomycosis.
Treatment/ prophylaxis regimen	Fluconazole 400 mg or 800 mg.
Results	Of 39 patients evaluable for efficacy analysis, 34 (87%) were successfully treated, including 89% and 85% of patients who received 400 and 800 mg, respectively. Five (83%) of six patients for whom prior antifungal therapy had failed were successfully treated. The mean duration of therapy was 8.9 months for successfully treated patients. Nineteen patients (48%) reported adverse events, although most were minor.
Conclusion	The authors conclude that fluconazole at daily doses of 400–800 mg for at least 6 months is effective therapy for non-life-threatening blastomycosis.

2. Pathogens

d. Blastomycosis/ Histoplasmosis

Title	Itraconazole therapy for blastomycosis and histoplasmosis.
Authors	Dismukes WE, Bradsher RW Jr., Cloud GC, et al.
Reference	Am J Med 1992;93(5):489–497.
Disease/ Pathogen	Blastomycosis and histoplasmosis.
Purpose	To assess the efficacy and toxicity of orally administered itraconazole in the treatment of nonmeningeal, nonlife-threatening forms of blastomycosis and histoplasmosis.
Design	Prospective, nonrandomized, open, multicenter trial.
Patients	85 patients with culture or histopathologic evidence of blastomycosis (48 patients) or histoplasmosis (37 patients). Patients receiving other systemic antifungal therapy were excluded.
Follow-up	Disease activity was assessed at baseline; drug efficacy and toxicity were evaluated at monthly intervals during therapy, and efficacy was evaluated at regular follow-up visits after completion of therapy. The median duration of post-treatment evaluation for successfully treated patients was 11.9 months (blastomycosis) and 12.1 months (histoplasmosis).
Treatment/ prophylaxis regimen	Itraconazole was administered orally at doses of 200–400 mg/d. Patients in whom treatment was considered a success were treated for a median duration of 6.2 months (blastomycosis) and 9 months (histoplasmosis).

Results   Among the 48 patients with blastomycosis, success was documented in 43 (90%). The success rate for patients treated for more than 2 months was 95%. Among the 37 patients with histoplasmosis, success was documented in 30 (81%). The success rate for patients treated for more than 2 months was 86%. All patients with histoplasmosis, in whom treatment failed, had chronic cavitary pulmonary disease. Toxicity was minor; only 25 (29%) patients experienced any side effects, and itraconazole toxicity necessitated stopping therapy in only one patient.

Conclusion Itraconazole was a highly effective therapy for non-meningeal, nonlife-threatening blastomycosis and histoplasmosis. The drug was associated with minimal toxicity.

2. Pathogens

e. Brucellosis

Open, Randomized Therapeutic Trial of Six Antimicrobial Regimens in the Treatment of Human Brucellosis

Title	Open, randomized therapeutic trial of six antimicrobial regimens in the treatment of human brucellosis.
Authors	Montejo JM, Alberola I, Glez-Zarate P, et al.
Reference	Clin Infect Dis 1993;16(5):671–676.
Disease/ Pathogen	Brucellosis.
Purpose	To describe the results of six antimicrobial regimens used for the treatment of brucellosis.
Design	Randomized, open label study performed over two periods (1980–1983, and 1984–1987).
Treatment/ prophylaxis regimen	In the first period, rifampicin and doxycycline were used for 4 weeks, trimethoprim-sulfamethoxazole for 6 months, and doxycycline for 6 weeks. During the second period, we used streptomycin for 2 or 3 weeks together with doxycycline for 6 weeks and rifampicin with doxycycline for 6 weeks.
Results	Comparison of the results showed the following: (1) no statistically significant findings were revealed when the different regimens were compared; and (2) the regimens containing streptomycin yielded statistically more favorable results than those consisting of rifampicin and monotherapy when the patients treated with rifampicin were compared with those taking streptomycin and those receiving single-agent therapy.
Conclusion	No significant differences were observed between monotherapeutic regimens and those including rifampicin.

Treatment of Human Brucellosis with Doxycycline Plus Rifampin or Doxycycline Plus Streptomycin: A Randomized, Double Blind Study.

Title	Treatment of human brucellosis with doxycycline plus rifampin or doxycycline plus streptomycin: A randomized, double blind study.
Authors	Ariza J, Gudiol F, Pallares R, et al.
Reference	Ann Intern Med 1992;117(1):25–30.
Disease/ Pathogen	Brucellosis.
Purpose	To compare the effectiveness of doxycycline-rifampin (DR) combination therapy with that of the classic doxycycline-streptomycin (DS) combination in patients with brucellosis.
Design	A randomized, double blind study.
Patients	95 patients (68 men and 27 women; mean age, 39 years) diagnosed with brucellosis on the basis of both clinical and serologic findings; 81 of these patients had blood cultures positive for Brucella melitensis.
Follow-up	Therapeutic failure and relapse during the follow-up period (mean follow-up=15.7 months).
Treatment/ prophylaxis regimen	44 patients received doxycycline, 100 mg every 12 hours, and rifampin, 15 mg/kg body weight per day in a single morning dose, for 45 days; 51 patients received the same dose of doxycycline for 45 days plus streptomycin, 1 g/d for 15 days.

***Treatment of Human Brucellosis with Doxycycline
Plus Rifampin or Doxycycline Plus Streptomycin:
A Randomized, Double Blind Study.***

(continued)

Results
The mean time to defervescence was 4.2 days for the DR group and 3.2 days for the DS group (p>0.2). The actuarial probability of therapeutic failure or relapse at 12 months of follow-up (Kaplan-Meier) was 14.4% in the DR group and 5.9% in the DS group (difference 8.5%; 95% confidence interval [CI] -4.8%–21.6%; p>0.2). All three patients with spondylitis in the DR group failed therapy compared with one of four patients in the DS group. Excluding patients with spondylitis, the actuarial failure rate was 4.9% and 4.3% in the DR and DS groups, respectively, at 12 months of follow-up (difference 0.6%; CI -8.1%–9.4%; p>0.2).

Conclusion
Doxycycline-rifampin combination therapy for 45 days is as effective as the classic DS combination in most patients with brucellosis. However, DR therapy might be less effective in those patients with spondylitis.

2. Pathogens

f. Candidiasis

Ingestion of Yogurt Containing Lactobacillus Acidophilus as Prophylaxis for Candidal Vaginitis

Title	Ingestion of yogurt containing Lactobacillus acidophilus as prophylaxis for candidal vaginitis.
Authors	Hilton E, Isenberg HD, Alperstein P, et al.
Reference	Ann Intern Med 1992;116:353–357.
Disease/ Pathogen	Vulvovaginal candidal yeast infections.
Purpose	To assess whether daily ingestion of yogurt containing Lactobacillus acidophilus prevents vulvovaginal candidal infections.
Design	Crossover trial for at least 1 year, during which patients were examined for candidal infections and colonizations while receiving either a yogurt-free or a yogurt-containing diet. Patients served as their own controls.
Patients	33 women with recurrent candidal vaginitis were eligible after recruitment from community practices and clinics and through advertising. 12 patients were eliminated for protocol violations. Of the remaining 21 patients, eight, who were assigned to the yogurt arm, initially refused to enter the control phase 6 months later. Thus, 13 patients completed the protocol.
Follow-up	Colonization of lactobacilli and candida in the vagina and rectum; candidal infections of the vagina.
Treatment/ prophylaxis regimen	Women ate yogurt for 6 months of the study period.

Ingestion of Yogurt Containing *Lactobacillus Acidophilus* as Prophylaxis for Candidal Vaginitis

(continued)

Results
: 33 eligible patients were studied. A threefold decrease in infections was seen when patients consumed yogurt containing L. acidophilus. The mean (±SD) number of infections per 6 months was 2.54±1.66 in the control arm and 0.38±0.51 per 6 months in the yogurt arm (p=0.001). Candidal colonization decreased from a mean of 3.23±2.17 per 6 months in the control arm to 0.84±0.90 per 6 months in the yogurt arm (p=0.001).

Conclusion
: Daily ingestion of 8 ounces of yogurt containing L. acidophilus decreased both candidal colonization and infection.

A Randomized, Double Blind Comparison of Itraconazole Oral Solution and Fluconazole Tablets in the Treatment of Esophageal Candidiasis

Title	A randomized, double blind comparison of itraconazole oral solution and fluconazole tablets in the treatment of esophageal candidiasis.
Authors	Wilcox CM, Darouiche RO, Laine L, et al.
Reference	J Infect Dis 1997;176(1):227–232.
Disease/ Pathogen	Esophageal candidiasis.
Purpose	To compare the efficacy and safety of itraconazole oral solution and fluconazole tablets in the treatment of esophageal candidiasis.
Design	Multicenter, randomized, double blind study.
Patients	126 immunocompromised patients with esophageal candidiasis.
Follow-up	Severity of symptoms was assessed weekly during treatment and every 2 weeks during follow-up.
Treatment/ prophylaxis regimen	Patients were treated with itraconazole oral solution or fluconazole tablets (both at 100–200 mg) once daily for 3–8 weeks, for 2 weeks beyond the resolution of symptoms, and were then followed for 4 more weeks.

A Randomized, Double Blind Comparison of Itraconazole Oral Solution and Fluconazole Tablets in the Treatment of Esophageal Candidiasis

(continued)

Results | Patients treated with itraconazole oral solution had a rate of clinical response (cured or improved) comparable to that of patients treated with fluconazole (94% vs 91%). The mycologic eradication rate was 92% for itraconazole, and 78% for fluconazole. Both treatments were well tolerated.

Conclusion | Results from treatment with once-daily itraconazole oral solution was clinically comparable to those with fluconazole, and is an alternative for the treatment of esophageal candidiasis in immunocompromised patients.

Intravascular Catheter Exchange and Duration of Candidemia

Title	Intravascular catheter exchange and duration of candidemia.
Authors	Rex JH, Bennett JE, Sugar AM, et al.
Reference	Clin Infect Dis 1995;21(4):994-996.
Disease/ Pathogen	Candidemia.
Purpose	To compare amphoteracin B with fluconazole for the treatment of candidemia in nonneutropenic patients.
Design	Data on the management of intravascular catheters were collected.
Patients	Complete records were available for 91% of the 206 study patients.
Results	For the subset of patients with a catheter in place at the time of their first positive blood culture, removal and replacement of all intravascular catheters without exchange over a guidewire from a pre-existing line on or before the first day the study drug was administered were associated with a reduction in the subsequent mean duration ($\pm$SE) of candidemia, from 5.6$\pm$0.8 days to 2.6 $\pm$0.5 days (p<0.001).

Randomized Trial of Fluconazole Vs Nystatin for the Prophylaxis of Candida Infection Following Liver Transplantation

Title	Randomized trial of fluconazole vs nystatin for the prophylaxis of Candida infection following liver transplantation.
Authors	Lumbreras C, Cuervas-Mons V, Jara P, et al.
Reference	J Infect Dis 1996;174(3):583–588.
Disease/ Pathogen	Candida infection.
Purpose	To examine the safety and efficacy of fluconazole therapy for prevention of Candida infection in patients undergoing liver transplantation.
Design	Prospective, randomized, multicenter study addressed the safety and efficacy of fluconazole therapy in patients undergoing liver transplantation.
Patients	143 liver transplant patients.
Treatment/ prophylaxis regimen	76 patients received daily oral fluconazole (100 mg), and 67 received nystatin (4 x 10[6] U) during the first 28 days after transplantation.

Randomized Trial of Fluconazole Vs Nystatin for the Prophylaxis of Candida Infection Following Liver Transplantation

(continued)

Results   Candida colonization occurred in 25% and 53% of patients in the fluconazole and nystatin groups, respectively (p=0.04); 13% and 34% of patients in the respective groups had Candida infections (p=0.022). Of these patients, 10.5% in the fluconazole group, and 25.3% in the nystatin group, had superficial candidal infections (p=0.024). Invasive candidiasis developed in two patients in the fluconazole group (2.6%) and six in the nystatin group (9%) (p=0.12). There was no increased hepatotoxicity, cyclosporine interaction, or emergence of clinically relevant resistant Candida strains attributable to fluconazole.

Conclusion   Oral fluconazole (100 mg) is safe and reduces Candida colonization and infection after liver transplantation.

A Randomized Trial Comparing Fluconazole with Amphotericin B for the Treatment of Candidemia in Patients Without Neutropenia

Title	A randomized trial comparing fluconazole with amphotericin B for the treatment of candidemia in patients without neutropenia.
Authors	Rex JH, Bennett JE, Sugar AM, et al.
Reference	N Engl J Med 1994;331(20):1325–1330.
Disease/ Pathogen	Candidemia.
Purpose	To compare amphotericin B with fluconazole as treatment for candidemia.
Design	Multicenter, randomized trial.
Patients	To be eligible, patients had to have a positive blood culture for Candida species, a neutrophil count ≥500 per cubic millimeter, and no major immunodeficiency. Of the 237 patients enrolled, 206 met all entry criteria.
Treatment/ prophylaxis regimen	Patients were randomly assigned to receive either amphotericin B (0.5–0.6 mg per kilogram of body weight per day) or fluconazole (400 mg per day). Each continued for at least 14 days after the last positive blood culture.

A Randomized Trial Comparing Fluconazole with Amphotericin B for the Treatment of Candidemia in Patients Without Neutropenia

(continued)

Results
The most common diagnoses were renal failure, non-hematologic cancer, and gastrointestinal disease. There was no statistically significant difference in outcome: Of the 103 patients treated with amphotericin B, 81 (79%) were judged to have been treated successfully, as were 72 of the 103 patients treated with fluconazole (70% p=0.22; 95% confidence interval [CI] for the difference, -5%–23%). The bloodstream infection failed to clear in 12 patients in the amphotericin group, and 15 in the fluconazole group; the species most commonly associated with failure was Candida albicans. There were 41 deaths in the amphotericin group, and 34 deaths in the fluconazole group (p=0.20). Intravascular catheters appeared to be the most frequent source of candidemia. There was less toxicity with fluconazole that with amphotericin B.

Conclusion
In patients without neutropenia and without major immunodeficiency, fluconazole and amphotericin B are not significantly different in their effectiveness in treating candidemia.

2. Pathogens

g. Chancroid

Comparison of Azithromycin and Ceftriaxone for the Treatment of Chancroid

Title	Comparison of azithromycin and ceftriaxone for the treatment of chancroid.
Authors	Martin DH, Sargent SJ, Wendel GD Jr., et al.
Reference	Clin Infect Dis. 21(2):409–14, 1995 Aug.
Disease/ Pathogen	Haemophilus ducreyi.
Purpose	To determine the efficacy of single-dose azithromycin for the treatment of chancroid.
Design	Randomized, unblinded, prospective study.
Patients	Men and women 16 years of age and older, who had dark-field-negative genital ulcers that were clinically suspected to be caused by H. ducreyi and who attended urban sexually transmitted disease clinics or presented to hospital emergency departments, were enrolled in the study.
Follow-up	Patients were followed for up to 23 days after treatment.
Treatment/ prophylaxis regimen	Patients were randomized to receive 250 mg of ceftriaxone intramuscular or 1 g of azithromycin orally, both given as a single dose.

Results	For 65 patients, cultures were positive for H. ducreyi. There were 68 patients whose cultures were negative for both H. ducreyi and herpes simplex virus, and who had no evidence of syphilis. All 133 patients returned for at least one follow-up visit. At the time of the last follow-up visit, all 32 patients whose cultures were positive for H. ducreyi, and who were treated with azithromycin, were clinically cured. In all 33 culture-positive cases in which ceftriaxone was used, there was either clinical improvement or cure at the time of the patient's last follow-up visit. In addition, azithromycin and ceftriaxone were equally effective in healing ulcers for which cultures were negative.
Conclusion	A single 1-g oral dose of azithromycin is as effective as a 250-mg intramuscular dose of ceftriaxone for the treatment of chancroid.

2. Pathogens

h. Chlamydial Infections

Randomised Comparison of Amoxycillin and Erythromycin in Treatment of Genital Chlamydial Infections in Pregnancy

Title	Randomised comparison of amoxycillin and erythromycin in treatment of genital chlamydial infections in pregnancy.
Authors	Alary M, Joly JR, Moutquin JM, et al.
Reference	Lancet 1994;344:1461–1465.
Disease/ Pathogen	Chlamydia.
Purpose	To compare amoxycillin with erythromycin for the treatment of chlamydial infection in pregnant women.
Design	Randomized, double blind trial.
Patients	210 pregnant women with Chlamydia trachomatis infection.
Follow-up	Control cultures were obtained 21 days after treatment, during late pregnancy, and from the infant within a week of birth. Treatment was judged a failure if any post-treatment culture was positive or if the patient had to stop therapy because of severe side-effects.
Treatment/ prophylaxis regimen	Pregnant women with C. trachomatis infection were randomly assigned 7 days' treatment with amoxycillin (500 mg three times daily) or erythromycin (500 mg four times daily).

Results   11 women (5.2%) were lost to follow-up. One (of 100) amoxycillin-treated women had to stop treatment because of severe side-effects, compared with 12 (of 99) erythromycin-treated women (p=0.002). one woman in the amoxycillin group had a positive culture at the third-trimester examination. No positive post-treatment culture was found in the erythromycin group. Severe gastrointestinal side-effects were more common in women who received erythromycin (31% vs 6%, p<0.001). The overall failure rate was therefore 2% in the amoxycillin group, and 12% in the erythromycin group (p=0.005).

Conclusion   These results suggest that amoxycillin is an acceptable alternative to erythromycin for C. trachomatis infection in pregnant women.

A Comparison of Oral Azithromycin with Topical Oxytetracycline/Polymyxin for the Treatment of Trachoma in Children

Title	A comparison of oral azithromycin with topical oxytetracycline/polymyxin for the treatment of trachoma in children.
Authors	Dawson CR, Schachter J, Sallam S, et al.
Reference	Clin Infect Dis 1997;24(3):363–368.
Disease/ Pathogen	Trachoma.
Purpose	To compare oral azithromycin with oxytetracycline/polymyxin eye ointment (once daily for 5 days every 4 weeks; total of six treatment cycles) for the treatment of active endemic trachoma in 168 rural Egyptian children.
Design	Randomized, prospective trial.
Patients	168 rural Egyptian children with endemic Chlamydia trachoma.
Follow-up	The children's clinical status and chlamydial infection rates were evaluated for 1 year.
Treatment/ prophylaxis regimen	A suspension of azithromycin was administered to children as a dose of 20 mg/kg by one of three schedules: A single dose, one dose a week for 3 weeks, and one dose every 4 weeks for a total of six doses.

A Comparison of Oral Azithromycin with Topical Oxytetracycline/Polymyxin for the Treatment of Trachoma in Children

Results   The clinical cure rates were 35% at 2 months after initial treatment, 16% at 8 months (during the annual autumn epidemic of purulent conjunctivitis), and 47% at 1 year. The pretreatment chlamydial infection rate of 33% (determined by direct immunofluorescence) decreased to 5% at 2 months and was 9% at 12 months. There were no significant clinical or laboratory differences among the four treatment groups.

Conclusion   Thus, 1-6 doses of azithromycin were equivalent to 30 days of topical oxytetracycline/polymyxin ointment and may offer an effective alternative means of controlling endemic trachoma.

Ciprofloxacin Compared with Doxycycline for Nongonococcal Urethritis: Ineffectiveness Against Chlamydia Trachomatis Due to Relapsing Infection.

Title	Ciprofloxacin compared with doxycycline for nongonococcal urethritis: Ineffectiveness against Chlamydia trachomatis due to relapsing infection.
Authors	Hooton TM, Rogers ME, Medina TG, et al.
Reference	JAMA 1990;264:1418–1421.
Disease/ Pathogen	Nongonococcal urethritis.
Purpose	To determine the effectiveness of ciprofloxacin for chlamydial urethritis in men.
Design	Prospective, randomized, double blind trial.
Patients	178 men with nongonococcal urethritis.
Treatment/ prophylaxis regimen	7-day regimens of ciprofloxacin in dosages of 750 and 1000 mg twice daily with doxycycline 100 mg twice daily.
Results	The overall clinical response was comparable in the three treatment groups at both 2 and 4 weeks after therapy. However, among patients who initially had cultures positive for chlamydia, C. trachomatis was re-isolated within 4 weeks after treatment in none of 10 doxycycline-treated patients, in 11 (52%) of 21 patients treated with 750 mg of ciprofloxacin twice daily, and in six (38%) of 16 patients treated with 1000 mg of ciprofloxacin twice daily. Each of the recurrent strains was identical in serotype to the original infecting strain.

Ciprofloxacin Compared with Doxycycline for Nongonococcal Urethritis: Ineffectiveness Against Chlamydia Trachomatis Due to Relapsing Infection.

(continued)

Conclusion   Ciprofloxacin in dosages as high as 2 g daily is inadequate for treatment of chlamydial urethritis in men, often resulting in relapsing infections.

Randomised, Controlled Trial of Single-Dose Azithromycin in Treatment of Trachoma

Title	Randomised, controlled trial of single-dose azithromycin in treatment of trachoma.
Authors	Bailey RL, Arullendran P, Whittle HC, et al.
Reference	Lancet 1993;342:453–456.
Disease/ Pathogen	Trachoma.
Purpose	To assess the efficacy of azithromycin for the treatment of trachoma.
Design	Randomised, single-blind comparison.
Patients	194 patients with trachoma.
Follow-up	The patients were followed up for 26 weeks from the start of treatment by an observer unaware of treatment allocation.
Treatment/ prophylaxis regimen	Azithromycin (a single oral dose of 20 mg/kg) with conventional treatment (6 weeks of topical tetracycline plus erythromycin for severe cases) in two villages with endemic trachoma in Gambia.
Results	By 6 months' follow-up, trachoma had resolved in 76 (78%) of 97 subjects who received azithromycin, compared with 70 (72%) of 97 who were treated conventionally (95% confidence interval [CI] for difference -6%–18%). Compliance with both treatments was good, but that for conventional treatment could probably not be achieved outside the research setting. There were no significant differences in treatment effect, baseline characteristics, or re-emergent disease between the treatment groups.

Conclusion   Azithromycin was well tolerated. As a systemic treatment effective in a single dose, it has important potential for trachoma control.

Title	Prevention of pelvic inflammatory disease by screening for cervical chlamydial infection.
Authors	Scholes D, Stergachis A, Heidrich FE, et al.
Reference	N Engl J Med 1996;334:1362–1366.
Disease/ Pathogen	Pelvic inflammatory disease.
Purpose	To evaluate whether the use of these criteria to select women to be tested for cervical chlamydial infection would reduce the incidence of pelvic inflammatory disease (PID).
Design	Randomized, controlled intervention trial.
Patients	2607 women, who were at high risk for disease, were identified by a questionnaire mailed to women enrollees in a health maintenance organization, and 18–34 years of age.
Follow-up	12 month follow-up.
Treatment/ prophylaxis regimen	Eligible respondents were randomly assigned to undergo testing for Chlamydia trachomatis or to receive usual care; both groups were followed for 1 year.

(continued)

Results	Of the 2607 eligible women, 1009 were randomly assigned to screening, and 1598 to usual care. A total of 645 women in the screening group (64 %) were tested for chlamydia; 7% tested positive and were treated. At the end of the follow-up period, there had been nine verified cases of PID among the women in the screening group, and 33 cases among the women receiving usual care (relative risk 0.44; 95% confidence interval 0.2–0.9). The authors found similar results when they used logistic-regression analysis to control for potentially confounding variables.
Conclusion	A strategy of identifying, testing, and treating women at increased risk for cervical chlamydial infection was associated with a reduced incidence of PID.

Chronic Chlamydia Pneumoniae Infection as a Risk Factor for Coronary Heart Disease in the Helsinki Heart Study

Title	Chronic Chlamydia pneumoniae infection as a risk factor for coronary heart disease in the Helsinki Heart Study.
Authors	Saikku P, Leinonen M, Tenkanen L, et al.
Reference	Ann Intern Med 1992;116:273–278.
Disease/ Pathogen	Chlamydia pneumoniae infection.
Purpose	To investigate in the prospective Helsinki Heart Study, whether chronic C. pneumoniae infection, indicated by elevated antibody titers against the pathogen, chlamydial lipopolysaccharide-containing immune complexes, or both, is a risk factor for coronary heart disease.
Design	The Helsinki Heart Study was a randomized, double blind, 5-year clinical trial to test the efficacy of gemfibrozil in reducing the risk for coronary heart disease.
Patients	140 cardiac events occurred during the follow-up period. Serum samples from 103 case patients obtained 3–6 months before a cardiac end point were matched with those from controls for time point, locality, and treatment. Samples were tested for markers of chronic chlamydial infection.

Chronic Chlamydia Pneumoniae Infection as a Risk Factor for Coronary Heart Disease in the Helsinki Heart Study

(continued)

Follow-up	Fatal and nonfatal myocardial infarction and sudden cardiac death were the main study end points. Serum samples were collected at 3-month intervals from all patients. Immunoglobulin A (IgA) and G (IgG) antibodies to C. pneumoniae were measured using the micro-immunofluorescence method. Lipopolysaccharide-containing immune complexes were measured using two antigen-specific enzyme immuno-assays, the lipopolysaccharide-capture and immunoglobulin M (IgM)-capture methods.
Treatment/ prophylaxis regimen	Participants were randomized to receive either gemfibrozil (2046 patients) or placebo (2035 patients).
Results	Using a conditional logistic regression model, odds ratios for the development of coronary heart disease were 2.7 (95% confidence interval [CI] 1.1-6.5) for elevated IgA titers, 2.1 (CI 1.1-3.9) for the presence of immune complexes, and 2.9 (CI 1.5-5.4) for the presence of both factors. If we adjusted for other coronary heart disease risk factors such as age, hypertension, and smoking, the corresponding values would be 2.3 (CI 0.9-6.2), 1.8 (CI 0.9-3.6), and 2.6 (CI 1.3-5.2), respectively.
Conclusion	The results suggest that chronic C. pneumoniae infection may be a significant risk factor for the development of coronary heart disease.

2. Pathogens

i. Clostridium Difficile Infections

Treatment of Asymptomatic Clostridium Difficile Carriers (Fecal Excretors) with Vancomycin or Metronidazole: A Randomized, Placebo Controlled Trial.

Title	Treatment of asymptomatic Clostridium difficile carriers (fecal excretors) with vancomycin or metronidazole: A randomized, placebo controlled trial.
Authors	Johnson S, Homann SR, Bettin KM, et al.
Reference	Ann Intern Med 1992;117(4):297–302.
Disease/ Pathogen	Clostridium difficile.
Purpose	To compare the efficacy of vancomycin and metronidazole for eradication of asymptomatic C. difficile fecal excretion as a means of controlling nosocomial outbreaks of C. difficile diarrhea.
Design	Randomized, placebo controlled, nonblinded trial.
Patients	30 patients excreting C. difficile without diarrhea or abdominal symptoms.
Follow-up	Stool cultures were obtained during treatment and for 2 months after treatment. All C. difficile isolates were typed by restriction endonuclease analysis (REA).
Treatment/ prophylaxis regimen	All patients were randomized to receive 10 days of oral vancomycin, 125 mg four times daily; metronidazole, 500 mg twice daily; or placebo, three times daily.

Treatment of Asymptomatic Clostridium Difficile Carriers (Fecal Excretors) with Vancomycin or Metronidazole: A Randomized, Placebo Controlled Trial.

(continued)

Results

C. difficile organisms were not detected during and immediately after treatment in nine of 10 patients treated with vancomycin, compared with three of 10 patients treated with metronidazole (p=0.02), and two of 10 patients in the placebo group (p=0.005). The fecal vancomycin concentration was 1406±1164 micrograms/g feces, but metronidazole was not detectable in nine of 10 patients. Eight of the nine evaluable patients who had negative stool cultures after treatment with vancomycin began to excrete C. difficile again 20±8 days after completing treatment. Three of these patients received additional antibiotics before C. difficile excretion recurred, and five acquired new C. difficile REA strains. Four of six patients who received only vancomycin before C. difficile excretion recurred were culture-positive at the end of the study compared with one of nine patients who received only placebo (p=0.047).

Conclusion

Asymptomatic fecal excretion of C. difficile is transient in most patients, and treatment with metronidazole is not effective. Although treatment with vancomycin is temporarily effective, it is associated with a significantly higher rate of C. difficile carriage 2 months after treatment and is not recommended.

Empiric Treatment of Acute Diarrheal Disease with Norfloxacin: A Randomized, Placebo Controlled Study. Swedish Study Group.

Title	Empiric treatment of acute diarrheal disease with norfloxacin: A randomized, placebo controlled study. Swedish Study Group.
Authors	Wistrom J, Jertborn M, Ekwall E, et al.
Reference	Ann Intern Med 1992;117(3):202–208.
Disease/ Pathogen	Acute diarrheal disease.
Purpose	To evaluate the clinical and microbiologic efficacy and safety of norfloxacin for acute diarrhea.
Design	Double blind, placebo controlled, randomized, clinical, multicenter trial.
Patients	Patients 12 years of age or older, with a history of acute diarrhea lasting 5 or fewer days. Eighty-five percent of patients (511/598) were evaluable for efficacy. Of these evaluable patients, 70% had traveled abroad within the previous 6 weeks.
Follow-up	Enteric pathogens were isolated in 51% of the evaluable patients: Campylobacter species in 29%, Salmonella species in 16%, Shigella species in 3.5%, and other pathogens in 2.6%.
Treatment/ prophylaxis regimen	Patients received either norfloxacin, 400 mg, or placebo twice daily for 5 days.

Empiric Treatment of Acute Diarrheal Disease with Norfloxacin: A Randomized, Placebo Controlled Study. Swedish Study Group.

(continued)

Results

Norfloxacin had a favorable overall effect, compared with placebo (cure rate 63%, compared with 51%; p=0.003). There were statistically favorable effects in culture-positive patients, patients with salmonellosis, and severely ill patients, but not in culture-negative patients or patients with campylobacteriosis or shigellosis. A significant difference was noted between norfloxacin and placebo in median time to cure among all evaluable patients (3, compared with 4 days; p=0.02) and in patients with campylobacteriosis (3, compared with 5 days; p=0.05) but not in patients. Culture-positive, but not culture-negative patients, in the norfloxacin group, had significantly fewer loose stools per day, compared with patients in the placebo group from day 2 onward (p≤0.01). Norfloxacin was significantly less effective than placebo in eliminating Salmonella species on days 12-17 (18%, compared with 49%; p=0.006), whereas the opposite was true for Campylobacter species (70%, compared with 50%, p=0.03). In six of nine patients tested, norfloxacin-resistant Campylobacter species (MIC, ≥32 micrograms/mL) appeared after norfloxacin treatment.

Conclusion

Empiric treatment reduced the intensity and, to some extent, the duration of symptoms of acute diarrhea. The effect was restricted to patients who had bacterial enteropathogens or who were severely ill. The clinical usefulness of this treatment is limited by the fact that norfloxacin seems to delay the elimination of salmonella and to induce resistance in campylobacter.

2. Pathogens

j. Coccidioidomycosis

Fluconazole in the Treatment of Chronic Pulmonary and Nonmeningeal Disseminated Coccidioidomycosis

Title	Fluconazole in the treatment of chronic pulmonary and nonmeningeal disseminated coccidioidomycosis.
Authors	Catanzaro A, Galgiani JN, Levine BE, et al.
Reference	Am J Med 1995;98(3):249–256.
Disease/ Pathogen	Nonmeningeal disseminated coccidioidomycosis.
Purpose	To determine the efficacy and safety of fluconazole as treatment for coccidioidomycosis.
Design	Multicenter, open label, single arm study.
Patients	Of 78 patients enrolled, 22 had soft-tissue, 42 had chronic pulmonary, and 14 had skeletal coccidioidomycosis. 49 had at least one concomitant disease, 7 of whom had human immunodefficiency virus infection.
Follow-up	Predefined assessment of disease-related abnormalities was performed at the time of enrollment, and repeated at least every 4 months. A satisfactory response was defined as any reduction of baseline abnormality by month 4, and at least 51% reduction by month 8.
Treatment/ prophylaxis regimen	Patients were given oral fluconazole 200 mg/d. Nonresponders were increased to 400 mg/d. Treatment courses were long: A mean of 323±230 days at 200 mg and 433±178 days at 400 mg.

Results   Among 75 evaluable patients, a satisfactory response was observed in 12 (86%) of the 14 patients with skeletal, 22 (55%) of the 40 patients with chronic pulmonary, and 16 (76%) of the 21 patients with soft-tissue disease. Five patients (7%) required modification of treatment due to toxicity. 41 patients who responded were followed off drug. 15 (37%) of them experienced reactivation of infection.

Conclusion   Fluconazole 200 or 400 mg/d is well tolerated and a moderately effective treatment for chronic pulmonary or nonmeningeal disseminated coccidioidomycosis. The relapse rate following therapy is high. Treatment trials with higher doses appear warranted. The relative efficacy of fluconazole vs other azoles or amphotericin B remains unknown.

Title	Fluconazole therapy for coccidioidal meningitis.
Authors	Galgiani JN, Catanzaro A, Cloud GA et al.
Reference	Ann Intern Med 1993;119(1):28–35.
Disease/ Pathogen	Coccidioidal meningitis.
Purpose	To determine the efficacy and safety of fluconazole treatment of coccidioidal meningitis.
Design	Uncontrolled, clinical trial.
Patients	50 consecutive patients with active coccidioidal meningitis, of whom 47 (94%) were evaluable. 25 patients had received no previous treatment for their meningitis, and nine had co-infection with human immunodeficiency virus (HIV).
Follow-up	Predefined assessment of infection-related abnormalities was done at the time of enrollment and was repeated at least every 4 months during treatment. Elimination of 40% or more of baseline abnormalities was considered a response.
Treatment/ prophylaxis regimen	Fluconazole was administered in an oral dose of 400 mg once per day, for up to 4 years (median, 37 months) in responding patients. Concurrent therapy with another antifungal agent was prohibited.

Results
37 of 47 (79%; 95% confidence interval 61%–90%) evaluable patients responded to treatment. Response rates were similar for patients with and without previous therapy, for patients with and without concomitant HIV infection, and for patients with and without pre-existing hydrocephalus. Most improvement occurred within 4–8 months after starting treatment. Patient symptoms resolved more quickly than did cerebrospinal fluid abnormalities. In 15 of 20 resonding patients followed for 20 months or more, residual low-level cerebrospinal fluid abnormalities remained throughout therapy. No patient discontinued therapy because of drug-related side effects, although confusion developed in two patients that resolved when the dose of fluconazole was reduced.

Conclusion
Fluconazole therapy is often effective in suppressing coccidioidal menigitis.

2. Pathogens

k. Condylomata Acuminata

A Randomized, Double Blind, Placebo Controlled Trial of Systemically Administered Interferon-Alpha, -Beta, or -Gamma in Combination with Cryotherapy for the Treatment of Condylomata Acuminatum

Title	A randomized, double blind, placebo controlled trial of systemically administered interferon-alpha, -beta, or -gamma in combination with cryotherapy for the treatment of condylomata acuminatum.
Authors	Bonnez W, Oakes D, Bailey-Farchione A, et al.
Reference	J Infect Dis 1995;171(5):1081–1089.
Disease/ Pathogen	Condyloma acuminata.
Purpose	To evaluate three interferon (IFN) preparations used in combination with cryotherapy for treatment of anogenital warts.
Design	Randomized, double blind, placebo controlled trial.
Patients	152 patients with condyloma acuminata.
Follow-up	Subjects were followed ≤1 year.
Treatment/ prophylaxis regimen	Subjects received subcutaneous injections (2×10^6 units/m^2) of IFN-alpha, -beta, -gamma or placebo three times a week for 6 weeks and cryotherapy with liquid nitrogen.

A Randomized, Double Blind, Placebo Controlled Trial of Systemically Administered Interferon-Alpha, -Beta, or -Gamma in Combination with Cryotherapy for the Treatment of Condylomata Acuminatum

(continued)

Results	Among patients followed ≥12 weeks, two thirds had a complete response. No significant differences in rates of complete response (p=0.37) or reappearance of a wart at the initial site (p=0.20) were noted among the treatment groups. However, patients who received IFN-beta or -gamma developed new warts at a significantly lower frequency (p=0.02).
Conclusion	IFN administration was associated with side effects, but was well tolerated. IFN-beta was the least toxic of the three preparations and had the best therapeutic ratio.

2. Pathogens

1. Cryptosporidiosis

Cryptosporidiosis: An Outbreak Associated with Drinking Water, Despite State-of-the-Art Water Treatment.

Title	Cryptosporidiosis: An outbreak associated with drinking water, despite state-of-the-art water treatment.
Authors	Goldstein ST, Juranek DD, Ravenholt O, et al.
Reference	Ann Intern Med 1996;124(5):459–468.
Disease/ Pathogen	Cryptosporidiosis.
Purpose	To determine the magnitude and source of an outbreak of crytosporidiosis among persons with human immunodeficiency virus (HIV) infection and to determine whether the outbreak extended into the immunocompetent population.
Design	Matched case-control study and environmental investigation.
Patients	Adults with HIV infection (36 case-patients with laboratory-confirmed Cryptosporidium parvum infection and 107 controls), matched by physician or clinic and by CD4+ cell count category.
Follow-up	Potential risk factors for infection, death rates, and data on water quality.

Cryptosporidiosis: An Outbreak Associated with Drinking Water, Despite State-of-the-Art Water Treatment.

(continued)

Results

Review of surveillance and microbiology records identified three cases of cryptosporidiosis in 1992 (the first year that cryptosporidiosis was reportable in Nevada), 23 cases in 1993, and 78 cases in the first quarter of 1994. Of the 78 laboratory-confirmed cases in the first quarter of 1994, 61 (78.2%) were in HIV-infected adults. Of these 61 adults, 32 (52.5%) had died by 30 June 1994; at least 20 of the 32 (62.5%) had cryptosporidiosis listed on their death certificates. In the case-control study, persons who drank only any unboiled tap water were four times more likely than persons who drank only bottled water to have had cryptosporidiosis (odd ratio 4.22 [95% confidence interval [CI] 1.22–14.65]; p=0.02). For persons, with CD4+ cell count less than 100 cell/mm^3, the association between tap water and cryptosporidiosis was even stronger (odds ratio 13.52 [CI 1.78–102.92]; p=0.01). Additional data indicate that this outbreak also affected persons who were not infected with HIV. No elevated turbidity values or coliform counts and no Cryptosporidium oocysts were found in testing of source (Lake Mead) or finished (treated) water during the study period, but so-called presumptive oocysts were intermittently found after the investigation in samples of souce water, filter backwash, and finished water.

Conclusion

A cryptosporidiosis outbreak was associated with municipal drinking water, despite state-of-the-art water treatment and water quality better than that required by current federal standards. This outbreak highlights the importance of surveillance for crypotosporidiosis and the need for guidelines for the prevention of water-borne-Cryprosporidium infection among HIV-infected persons.

2. Pathogens

m. Cyclosporidiosis

Placebo Controlled Trial of Co-Trimoxazole for Cyclospora Infections Among Travelers and Foreign Residents in Nepal

Title	Placebo controlled trial of co-trimoxazole for cyclospora infections among Travelers and foreign residents in Nepal.
Authors	Hoge CW, Shlim DR, Ghimire M, et al.
Reference	Lancet 1995;345:691–693.
Disease/ Pathogen	Cyclosporidiosis.
Purpose	To determine the effect of co-trimoxazole for cyclospora infections among travellers and foreign residents in Nepal.
Design	Randomised, double blinded trial.
Patients	40 patients.
Treatment/ prophylaxis regimen	Participants were assigned to receive either cotrimoxazole (160 mg trimethoprim, 800 mg sulphamethoxazole) or placebo tablets twice daily for 7 days. Of 40 patients included in the study, 21 received co-trimoxazole and 19 placebo.
Results	There were no significant differences between these two groups in age, sex, time in Nepal, duration, severity of illness, or presence of other enteric pathogens. After 3 days, 71% of patients receiving co-trimoxazole still had cyclospora detected, compared with 100% of patients receiving placebo (p=0.016). After 7 days, cyclospora was detected in one (6%) of 16 patients treated with co-trimoxazole who submitted stool specimens, compared with 15 (88%) of 17 patients receiving placebo (p<0.0001). Eradication of the organism was correlated with clinical improvement. There was no evidence of relapse of infection among treated patients followed for an additional 7 days.

Conclusion   Treatment with co-trimoxazole for 7 days was effective in curing cyclospora infection among an expatriate population in Nepal.

2. Pathogens

n. Cysticercosis

Title	Serologic evolution of neurocysticercosis patients after antiparasitic therapy.
Authors	Garcia HH, Gilman RH, Catacora M, et al.
Reference	J Infect Dis 1997;175(2):486–489.
Disease/ Pathogen	Neurocysticercosis.
Purpose	This study analyzed the relationship between clinical characteristics of cerebral infection (number and type of lesions) plus the baseline response on immunoblot and the changes observed after therapy.
Results	Reaction to all seven diagnostic bands was associated with severe infection (more lesions). 17 patients (35%) had no active lesions on computed tomography (CT) 3 months after therapy, and were considered cured. Although most cured patients remained seropositive after 1 year, three became seronegative before 9 months. In these three cases, the lesions had resolved on CT at 3 months.
Conclusion	Persistent seropositivity does not necessarily indicate active infection. Serologic follow-up will be clinically help-ful only in rare cases in which early antibody disappear-ance occurs.

2. Pathogens

o. Cytomegalovirus Infections

Randomised Trial of Efficacy and Safety of Oral Ganciclovir in the Prevention of Cytomegalovirus Disease in Liver-Transplant Recipients

Title	Randomised trial of efficacy and safety of oral ganciclovir in the prevention of cytomegalovirus disease in liver-transplant recipients.
Authors	Gane E, Saliba F, Valdecasas GJ, et al.
Reference	Lancet 1997;350:1729–1733.
Disease/ Pathogen	Cytomegalovirus (CMV) infection.
Purpose	To study the safety and efficacy of oral ganciclovir in the prevention of CMV disease following orthotopic liver transplantation.
Design	Randomized, placebo controlled.
Patients	304 liver-transplant recipients
Follow-up	Patients were assessed at specified times throughout the first 6 months after surgery for evidence of CMV infection, CMV disease, rejection, opportunistic infections, and possible drug toxicity.
Treatment/ prophylaxis regimen	Patients were randomized to receive oral ganciclovir 1000 mg or matching placebo three times a day.

(continued)

Results   The Kaplan-Meier estimate of the 6-month incidence of CMV disease was 29 (18.9%) of 154 in the placebo group, compared with seven (4.8%) of 150 in the ganciclovir group (p<0.001). In the high-risk group of seronegative recipients (R-) of seropositive livers (D+), incidence of CMV disease was 11 (44%) of 25 in the placebo group, three (14.8%) of 21 in the ganciclovir group (p=0.02). Significant benefit was also observed in those receiving antibodies to lymphocytes, where the incidence of CMV disease was 12 (32.9%) of 37 in the placebo group, and two (4.6%) of 44 in the ganciclovir group (p=0.002). Oral ganciclovir reduced the incidence of CMV infection (placebo 79 [51.5%] of 154; ganciclovir 37 [24.5%] of 150; p < 0.001) and also reduced symptomatic herpes-simplex infections (Kaplan-Meier estimates: Placebo 36 [23.5%] of 154; ganciclovir five [3.5%] of 150; p<0.001).

Conclusion   Oral ganciclovir is a safe and effective method for the prevention of CMV disease after orthotopic liver transplantation.

Impact of Long-Term Acyclovir on Cytomegalovirus Infection and Survival After Allogeneic Bone Marrow Transplantation

Title	Impact of long-term acyclovir on cytomegalovirus infection and survival after allogeneic bone marrow transplantation.
Authors	Prentice HG, Gluckman E, Powles RL, et al.
Reference	Lancet 1994;343:749–753.
Disease/ Pathogen	Cytomegalovirus (CMV) infection.
Purpose	To study the prophylactic effect of high-dose intravenous acyclovir given around the time of bone marrow transplant (BMT) followed by oral acyclovir on CMV infection and survival.
Design	Double blind, double dummy.
Patients	310 BMT recipients at risk of developing CMV infection were randomised to one of three regimens.
Treatment/ prophylaxis regimen	Intravenous acylclovir (500 mg/m^2, three times a day) for 1 month followed by oral acyclovir (800 mg four times a day for a further 6 months) (intravenous/oral group); intravenous acyclovir followed by oral placebo (intermediate group); or low-dose oral acyclovir (200 or 400 mg, four times a day) followed by placebo ("controls").

(continued)

Results	Intravenous acyclovir significantly reduced the probability of and delayed the onset of CMV infection. There was no further reduction in infection risk with the addition of long-term oral acyclovir. Time to CMV viraemia was delayed in the intravenous/oral acyclovir group compared with controls. Extending the prophylaxis with oral acyclovir significantly improved survival: 79 of 105 recipients were still alive at 7 months compared with 60 of 102 controls (p=0.012). Although the intravenous/oral acyclovir group did significantly better than controls in terms of survival, the difference between the intravenous/oral acyclovir group and the intermediate group was of borderline statistical significance (p=0.054). Adverse events that were possibly treatment-related were similar in all three groups. The most commonly reported events were nausea, vomiting, elevated creatinine, and renal failure.
Conclusion	High-dose intravenous followed by oral acyclovir improved survival and was of benefit in prophylaxis against the effects of CMV after BMT. Interpretation of CMV infection was made difficult because an intermediate treatment (intravenous acyclovir followed by oral placebo) was as effective as high-dose intravenous/oral acyclovir.

Ganciclovir Treatment of Symptomatic Congenital Cytomegalovirus Infection: Results of a Phase II Study.

Title	Ganciclovir treatment of symptomatic congenital cytomegalovirus infection: Results of a phase II study.
Authors	Whitley RJ, Cloud G, Gruber W, et al.
Reference	J Infect Dis 1997;175(5):1080–1086.
Disease/ Pathogen	Cytomegalovirus (CMV) infection.
Purpose	A phase II evaluation was done of ganciclovir for the treatment of symptomatic congenital CMV infection.
Design	Prospective study.
Patients	37 babies with congenital CMV infection.
Follow-up	Clinical and laboratory evaluations sought evidence of toxicity, quantitative virologic responses in urine, plasma drug concentrations, and clinical outcome.
Treatment/ prophylaxis regimen	Daily doses of 8 or 12 mg/kg were administered in divided doses at 12-hour intervals for 6 weeks.
Results	Significant laboratory abnormalities included thrombocytopenia ($\leq$50,000/mm^3) in 37 babies and absolute neutropenia ($\leq$500 mm^3) in 29 babies. Quantitative excretion of CMV in the urine decreased. However, after cessation of therapy, viruria returned to near pretreatment levels. Hearing improvement or stabilization occurred in 5 (16%) of 30 babies at 6 months or later, indicating efficacy.

Title	Valacyclovir for the prevention of cytomegalovirus disease after renal transplantation.
Authors	Lowance D, Neumayer HH, Legendre CM, et al.
Reference	N Engl J Med 1999;340:1462–1470.
Disease/ Pathogen	Cytomegalovirus (CMV) infection.
Purpose	To test whether valacyclovir is safe and efficacious as prophylaxis against CMV disease in recipients of renal allografts from cadaveric donors.
Design	Randomized, double blind, placebo controlled, multicenter.
Patients	A total of 208 CMV-negative recipients of a kidney from a seropositive donor and 408 CMV-positive recipients were randomly assigned to receive either 2 g of valacyclovir or placebo orally four times daily for 90 days after transplantation, with the dose adjusted according to renal function.
Follow-up	The efficacy of treatment was assessed for 6 months, and the safety of treatment and survival of patients and allografts were assessed for 1 year.

(continued)

Treatment/ prophylaxis regimen	Patients whose creatinine clearance exceeded 75 ml per minute received the 8 g dose, those with a creatinine clearance of 51-75 ml per minute received 6 g per day (1.5 g four times daily), those with a creatinine clearance of 26-50 ml per minute received 4.5 g per day (1.5 g three times daily), those with a creatinine clearance of 10-25 ml per minute received 3 g per day (1.5 g twice daily), and those who had a creatinine clearance of less than 10 ml per minute or who were on dialysis received 1.5 g per day.
Results	Treatment with valacyclovir reduced the incidence or delayed the onset of CMV disease in both the seronegative patients ($p<0.001$), and the seropositive patients ($p=0.03$). Among the seronegative patients, the incidence of CMV disease 90 days after transplantation was 45% among placebo recipients, and 3% among valacyclovir recipients. Among the seropositive patients, the respective values were 6% and 0%. At 6 months, the incidence of CMV disease was 45% among seronegative recipients of placebo and 16% among seronegative recipients of valacyclovir; it was 6 % among seropositive placebo recipients and 1% among seropositive valacyclovir recipients. At 6 months, the rate of biopsy-confirmed acute graft rejection in the seronegative group was 52% among placebo recipients, and 26% among valacyclovir recipients ($p=0.001$). Treatment with valacyclovir also decreased the rates of CMV viremia and viruria, herpes simplex virus disease, and the use of inpatient medical resources. Hallucinations and confusion were more common with valacyclovir treatment, but these events were not severe or treatment limiting. The rates of other adverse events were similar among the groups.
Conclusion	Prophylactic treatment with valacyclovir is a safe and effective way to prevent CMV disease after renal transplantation.

Pre-emptive Ganciclovir Therapy to Prevent Cytomegalovirus Disease in Cytomegalovirus Antibody-Positive Renal Transplant Recipients: A Randomized, Controlled Trial.

Title	Pre-emptive ganciclovir therapy to prevent cytomegalovirus disease in cytomegalovirus antibody-positive renal transplant recipients: A randomized, controlled trial.
Authors	Hibberd PL, Tolkoff-Rubin NE, Conti D, et al.
Reference	Ann Intern Med 1995;123:18–26.
Disease/ Pathogen	Cytomegalovirus (CMV) infection.
Purpose	To determine whether pre-emptive ganciclovir therapy administered daily during antilymphocyte antibody therapy can prevent CMV disease in renal transplant recipients who are positive for CMV antibody.
Design	Randomized, controlled, multicenter trial.
Patients	113 renal transplant recipients who were positive for CMV antibody.
Follow-up	6 months.
Treatment/ prophylaxis regimen	Patients were randomly assigned to receive either 1) ganciclovir, 2.5 mg/kg body weight administered intravenously on every day that antilymphocyte antibody therapy was administered; or 2) no anticytomegalovirus therapy.

Pre-emptive Ganciclovir Therapy to Prevent Cytomegalovirus Disease in Cytomegalovirus Antibody-Positive Renal Transplant Recipients: A Randomized, Controlled Trial.

(continued)

Results
CMV disease occurred in 14% of patients (9 of 64) who received pre-emptive ganciclovir therapy and in 33% of controls (16 of 49) (p=0.018). CMV was isolated from buffy-coat specimens from 17% of patients (11 of 64) receiving pre-emptive ganciclovir and from 35% of controls (17 of 49) (p=0.03). Controlling for the reason (induction or treatment of rejection) for using antilymphocyte antibodies in a Cox proportional hazards model, we found that pre-emptive ganciclovir still protected against CMV disease (adjusted relative risk 0.27; 95% confidence interval [CI] 0.12–0.64). No adverse events were attributed to pre-emptive ganciclovir therapy during or within 6 months of its administration.

Conclusion
Pre-emptive ganciclovir therapy administered daily during courses of treatment with antilymphocyte antibodies reduced the excessive occurrence of CMV disease in renal transplant recipients who were positive for CMV antibody. This approach, which links the most potent immunosuppression to intensive antimicrobial therapy, allows preventive therapy to be given to those patients at greatest risk for developing infectious complications. These patients are likely to benefit most from the preventive strategy.

High-Dose Acyclovir Compared with Short-Course Pre-emptive Ganciclovir Therapy to Prevent Cytomegalovirus Disease in Liver Transplant Recipients: A Randomized Trial.

Title	High-dose acyclovir compared with short-course pre-emptive ganciclovir therapy to prevent cytomegalovirus disease in liver transplant recipients: A randomized trial.
Authors	Singh N, Yu VL, Mieles L, et al.
Reference	Ann Intern Med 1994;120:375–381.
Disease/ Pathogen	Cytomegalovirus (CMV) infection.
Purpose	To assess the efficacy of high-dose oral acyclovir therapy compared with pre-emptive, short-course ganciclovir therapy (administered only if cytomegalovirus shedding occurred) to prevent CMV disease in liver transplant recipients.
Design	A randomized, controlled trial.
Patients	47 consecutive patients having liver transplantation.
Follow-up	24 weeks postoperatively.

High-Dose Acyclovir Compared with Short-Course Pre-emptive Ganciclovir Therapy to Prevent Cytomegalovirus Disease in Liver Transplant Recipients: A Randomized Trial.

(continued)

Treatment/ prophylaxis regimen	Patients were stratified by their CMV antibody status and the CMV antibody status of the donor and were randomly assigned to one of two treatment groups. Surveillance cultures for CMV (buffy coat and urine) were done every 2–4 weeks for 24 weeks in all patients. One group received high-dose oral acyclovir (800 mg four times daily). The experimental group received no acyclovir, but if surveillance cultures were positive, ganciclovir (5 mg/kg intravenously twice daily) was administered for 7 days.
Results	CMV shedding before the onset of CMV disease occurred in 25% (6 of 24) of patients in the acyclovir group compared with 22% (5 of 23) in the experimental group. CMV disease developed in 29% (7 of 24) of the acyclovir group and in 4% (1 of 23) of the experimental group (p<0.05). No hematologic toxicity occurred with ganciclovir.
Conclusion	Oral acyclovir is ineffective prophylaxis against CMV in liver transplant recipients. Pre-emptive, short-course ganciclovir therapy in patients with CMV shedding was well tolerated and provided effective prophylaxis against subsequent CMV disease. This protocol targets the patients at risk for CMV disease and minimizes toxicity and expense.

Title	Ganciclovir prophylaxis to prevent cytomegalovirus disease after allogeneic marrow transplant.
Authors	Goodrich JM, Bowden RA, Fisher L, et al.
Reference	Ann Intern Med 1993;118:173–178.
Disease/ Pathogen	Cytomegalovirus (CMV) infection.
Purpose	To study the efficacy and toxicity of ganciclovir prophylaxis given at engraftment to CMV-seropositive, allogeneic bone marrow transplant recipients.
Design	A double blind, placebo controlled study.
Patients	93 CMV-seropositive patients were entered into the study before marrow transplant, with 64 patients randomized to receive the study drug after marrow engraftment. 31 patients received placebo, and 33 received ganciclovir.
Follow-up	Outcome variables measured were CMV infection, monitored by weekly cultures, and neutropenia, defined as an absolute neutrophil count of 0.750 x 10-9/L for 2 consecutive days. Cytomegalovirus disease and mortality were secondary end points.
Treatment/ prophylaxis regimen	The ganciclovir dose was 5 mg/kg body weight administered intravenously twice daily for 5 days, followed by once daily until day 100 after transplant.

(continued)

Results   14 (45%) placebo recipients developed CMV infection in the first 100 days after marrow transplant compared with one (3%) ganciclovir recipient (p<0.001). Nine (29%) placebo recipients developed CMV disease, compared with no cases in the ganciclovir group during the first 100 days (p<0.001). Neutropenia occurred in 10 ganciclovir recipients (30%), compared with no cases in the placebo group during the period of observation (p=0.001). In a separate analysis, patients on ganciclovir who became neutropenic were at greater risk (relative risk 4.3; p=0.02) for bacterial infection. Mortality between the two study groups did not differ statistically at 100 and 180 days.

Conclusion   Ganciclovir given prophylactically after engraftment is effective in suppressing CMV infection and disease. Neutropenia is an important side effect of ganciclovir use and is associated with an increased risk for bacterial infection.

Ganciclovir Prophylaxis of Cytomegalovirus Infection and Disease in Allogeneic Bone Marrow Transplant Recipients: Results of a Placebo Controlled, Double Blind Trial.

Title	Ganciclovir prophylaxis of cytomegalovirus infection and disease in allogeneic bone marrow transplant recipients: Results of a placebo controlled, double blind trial.
Authors	Winston DJ, Ho WG, Bartoni K, et al.
Reference	Ann Intern Med 1993;118:179–184.
Disease/ Pathogen	Cytomegalovirus (CMV) infection.
Purpose	To evaluate the efficacy and safety of ganciclovir for prevention of CMV infection and disease.
Design	A randomized, placebo controlled, double blind trial.
Patients	CMV-seropositive allogeneic bone marrow transplant recipients.
Follow-up	CMV infection (positive culture, seroconversion, positive histologic findings), CMV disease (pneumonia, gastroenteritis, the wasting syndrome), and study-drug toxicity.
Treatment/ prophylaxis regimen	Random assignment to receive either a placebo or ganciclovir at a dose of 2.5 mg/kg body weight every 8 hours for 1 week before transplant and then at a dose of 6 mg/kg once per day, Monday through Friday, after transplant when the post-transplant neutrophil count reached 1 x 109/L.

Ganciclovir Prophylaxis of Cytomegalovirus Infection and Disease in Allogeneic Bone Marrow Transplant Recipients: Results of a Placebo Controlled, Double Blind Trial.

(continued)

Results

CMV infection developed in 25 of 45 placebo patients (56%) but in only eight of 40 ganciclovir patients (20%) ($p<0.001$). CMV disease may also have occurred less often in the ganciclovir patients (four of 40 patients (10%) vs 11 of 45 patients (24%); $p=0.09$). The probability of CMV disease occurring within the first 120 days after transplantation was 0.29 among the placebo patients, but only 0.12 among ganciclovir patients ($p=0.06$). Reversible neutropenia was the only appreciable toxicity related to ganciclovir and required interruption of the study drug after transplant in 25 of 43 ganciclovir patients (58%) and in 13 of 47 placebo patients (28%) ($p=0.005$). Overall survival was similar in both the placebo patients (29 of 45 (64%)) and ganciclovir patients (28 of 40 (70%); $p>0.2$).

Conclusion

Prophylactic ganciclovir, started before transplant and continued after recovery of the post-transplant neutrophil count, reduces the incidence and severity of CMV infection in CMV-seropositive bone marrow transplant recipients but is frequently associated with neutropenia.

A Controlled Trial of Ganciclovir to Prevent Cytomegalovirus Disease after Heart Transplantation

Title	A controlled trial of ganciclovir to prevent cytomegalovirus disease after heart transplantation.
Authors	Merigan TC, Renlund DG, Keay S, et al.
Reference	N Engl J Med 1992;326:1182–1186.
Disease/ Pathogen	Cytomegalovirus (CMV) infection.
Purpose	To evaluate the prophylactic administration of ganciclovir to prevent CMV-induced disease after heart transplantation.
Design	Randomized, double blind, placebo controlled, multicenter.
Patients	Patients seropositive for CMV before transplantation, and those who were seronegative, but who received hearts from seropositive donors.
Treatment/ prophylaxis regimen	Ganciclovir was given intravenously at a dose of 5 mg/kg of body weight every 12 hours from postoperative day 1–14, then at a dose of 6 mg/kg each day for 5 days per week until day 28.

Results

Among the seropositive patients, CMV illness occurred during the first 120 days after heart transplantation in 26 of 56 patients given placebo (46%), as compared with five of 56 patients treated with ganciclovir (9%) (p<0.001). Among 37 seronegative patients, CMV illness was frequent in both groups (placebo 29%; ganciclovir 35%; p not significant). From days 15–60, the patients who took ganciclovir had significantly fewer urine cultures positive for CMV, but by day 90 there was no difference. More of the ganciclovir-treated patients had serum creatinine concentrations greater than or equal to 221 mumol per liter (2.5 mg per deciliter) (18% vs 4% in the placebo group), but those elevations were transient.

Conclusion

The prophylactic administration of ganciclovir after heart transplantation is safe, and in CMV-seropositive patients it reduces the incidence of CMV-induced illness.

A Randomized, Controlled Trial of Prophylactic Ganciclovir for Cytomegalovirus Pulmonary Infection in Recipients of Allogeneic Bone Marrow Transplants

Title	A randomized, controlled trial of prophylactic ganciclovir for cytomegalovirus pulmonary infection in recipients of allogeneic bone marrow Transplants.
Authors	Schmidt GM, Horak DA, Niland JC, et al.
Reference	New Engl J Med 1991;324(15):1005–1011.
Disease/ Pathogen	Cytomegalovirus (CMV) infection.
Purpose	To conduct a controlled trial of ganciclovir in recipients of bone marrow transplants with asymptomatic pulmonary CMV infection and to identify risk factors for the development of CMV interstitial pneumonia.
Design	Randomized, controlled trial.
Patients	40 patients who had positive cultures for CMV were randomly assigned to either prophylactic ganciclovir or observation alone.
Treatment/ prophylaxis regimen	Ganciclovir (5 mg per kilogram of body weight intravenously) was given twice daily for two weeks and then five times per week until day 120.

A Randomized, Controlled Trial of Prophylactic Ganciclovir for Cytomegalovirus Pulmonary Infection in Recipients of Allogeneic Bone Marrow Transplants

(continued)

Results

Of the 20 culture-positive patients who received prophylactic ganciclovir, five (25%) died or had CMV pneumonia before day 120, as compared with 14 of the 20 culture-positive control patients (70%) who were not treated prophylactically (relative risk 0.36; p=0.01). No patient who received the full course of ganciclovir prophylaxis went on to have CMV interstitial pneumonia. Four patients treated with ganciclovir had maximal serum creatinine levels greater than or equal to 221 mumol per liter (2.5 mg per deciliter), as compared with none of the controls (p=0.029). Of the 55 CMV-negative patients who could be evaluated, 12 (22%) had CMV pneumonia—a significantly lower rate than in the untreated CMV-positive control patients (relative risk 0.33; p=0.003). The strongest predictors of CMV pneumonia were a lavage-fluid culture that was positive for CMV and a CMV-positive blood culture, both from specimens obtained on day 35.

Conclusion

In recipients of allogeneic bone marrow, asymptomatic CMV infection of the lung is a major risk factor for subsequent CMV interstitial pneumonia. Prophylactic ganciclovir is effective in preventing the development of CMV interstitial pneumonia in patients with asymptomatic infection.

Early Treatment with Ganciclovir to Prevent Cytomegalovirus Disease after Allogeneic Bone Marrow Transplantation

Title	Early treatment with ganciclovir to prevent cytomegalovirus disease after allogeneic bone marrow transplantation.
Authors	Goodrich JM, Mori M, Gleaves CA, et al,
Reference	New Engl J Med 1991;325:1601–1607.
Disease/ Pathogen	Cytomegalovirus (CMV) infection.
Purpose	To determine the effects of ganciclovir for the early treatment of CMV infection in asymptomatic recipients of bone marrow transplants whose surveillance cultures for CMV became positive.
Design	Double blind, controlled trial.
Patients	72 patients who had marrow engraftment and were excreting virus.
Follow-up	Patients were followed for the development of biopsy-confirmed CMV disease, ganciclovir-related toxicity, and survival.
Treatment/ prophylaxis regimen	Patients were randomly assigned to receive either placebo or ganciclovir (5 mg per kilogram of body weight twice a day for one week, followed by 5 mg per kilogram per day) for the first 100 days after transplantation.

Results

Between assignment to the study drug and day 100 after transplantation, CMV disease developed in only one of the 37 patients assigned to receive ganciclovir (3%), but in 15 of the 35 patients assigned to receive placebo (43%, $p<0.00001$). The ganciclovir recipients had rapid suppression of virus excretion; 85% had negative cultures after one week of treatment, as compared with 44% of the placebo group ($p=0.001$). The principal toxic reaction was neutropenia; 11 ganciclovir recipients had an absolute neutrophil count below $0.75 \times 10(9)$ per liter, as compared with three placebo recipients ($p=0.052$). Treatment was discontinued in 11 ganciclovir recipients and one placebo recipient because of neutropenia ($p=0.003$). After treatment was stopped, the neutrophil count recovered in all patients. Overall, survival was significantly greater in the ganciclovir group than in the placebo group both 100 days and 180 days after transplantation ($p=0.041$ and $0.02, 0.027$, respectively).

Conclusion

Early treatment with ganciclovir in patients with positive surveillance cultures reduces the incidence of CMV disease and improves survival after allogeneic bone marrow transplantation.

Randomized Comparison of Ganciclovir Plus Intravenous Immune globulin (IVIG) with IVIG Alone for Prevention of Primary Cytomegalovirus Disease in Children Receiving Liver Transplants

Title	Randomized comparison of ganciclovir plus intravenous immune globulin (IVIG) with IVIG alone for prevention of primary cytomegalovirus disease in children receiving liver transplants.
Authors	King SM, Superina R, Andrews W, et al.
Reference	Clin Infect Dis 1997;25(5):1173–1179.
Disease/ Pathogen	Cytomegalovirus (CMV) infection.
Purpose	To determine the benefit of ganciclovir for 30 days, in addition to intravenous immune globulin for 16 weeks for prevention of primary CMV disease in children receiving liver transplants.
Design	Randomized, placebo controlled trial.
Patients	56 children receiving liver transplants who were monitored for 6 months prior to surgery.
Treatment/ prophylaxis regimen	Patients received either ganciclovir (5 mg/[kg x d]) for 30 days, in addition to intravenous immune globulin (IVIG) for 16 weeks or placebo.

Randomized Comparison of Ganciclovir Plus Intravenous Immune globulin (IVIG) with IVIG Alone for Prevention of Primary Cytomegalovirus Disease in Children Receiving Liver Transplants

(continued)

Results

The two groups of patients (recipients of 29 ganciclovir plus IVIG and 27 recipients of IVIG alone) were similar in terms of age, sex, and underlying disease. The incidence of CMV disease among the ganciclovir plus IVIG recipients and the IVIG alone recipients was 17%, and 26%, respectively, and the time to disease in these recipients was 46 days, and 32 days, respectively. There was no difference between groups in terms of survival; episodes of rejection, bacteremia, or fungemia; use of immunosuppressive agents; and incidence of leukopenia or thrombocytopenia.

Conclusion

These results suggest that a 4-week course of ganciclovir with IVIG is not more effective than IVIG alone for prevention of primary CMV disease. Since short-term prophylaxis with ganciclovir may delay the onset of CMV disease, further studies with a longer course of ganciclovir prophylaxis are warranted.

2. Pathogens
p. Diphtheria

Title	Penicillin vs erythromycin in the treatment of diphtheria.
Authors	Kneen R, Pham NG, Solomon T, et al.
Reference	Clin Infect Dis 1998;27(4):845–850.
Disease/ Pathogen	Diphtheria.
Purpose	To compare penicillin with erythromycin in the treatment of Vietnamese children with diphtheria.
Design	Open label, randomized trial.
Patients	86 Vietnamese children with diphtheria.
Treatment/ prophylaxis regimen	44 children with diphtheria were given penicillin therapy (intramuscular benzylpenicillin, 50,000 U/[kg.d] for 5 days and then oral penicillin, 50 mg/[kg.d] for 5 days), and 42 were given erythromycin therapy (50 mg/[kg.d] orally for 10 days).

Results | There were no differences in times to membrane clearance or bacteriologic clearance, but median times to fever clearance were 27 hours (95% confidence interval [CI] 19–30; range 0-124 hours) for penicillin recipients and 46 hours (95% CI 34–54; range 0-148 hours) for erythromycin recipients (p=0.0004). In the penicillin group, acute treatment failed for one patient, and one patient relapsed. Three patients in the penicillin group developed diphtheritic myocarditis as evidenced by abnormal electrocardiograms. Erythromycin did not cause prolongation of the QT interval corrected for heart rate. Cultures of specimens from 15 patients (17.4%) were positive for toxigenic Corynebacterium diphtheriae. All isolates were susceptible to penicillin, but for isolates (27%), all of which were from patients who received penicillin treatment, were resistant to erythromycin (minimum inhibitory concentrations, >64 mg/L).

Conclusion | Penicillin is recommended as first-line treatment for diphtheria in Vietnam.

2. Pathogens

q. Echinococcosis

Percutaneous Drainage Compared with Surgery for Hepatic Hydatid Cysts

Title	Percutaneous drainage compared with surgery for hepatic hydatid cysts.
Authors	Khuroo MS, Wani NA, Javid G, et al.
Reference	N Engl J Med 1997;337:881–887.
Disease/ Pathogen	Echniococcosis.
Purpose	To compare percutaneous drainage with surgery in patients with hepatic hydatidosis.
Design	Prospective, randomized.
Patients	50 patients with hepatic hydatidosis.
Follow-up	Patient observed for 48 hours after surgery, and then discharged if there were no complications.
Treatment/ prophylaxis regimen	Simple cystectomy and drainage of the residual contents of the cyst cavity.

Results

The mean (±SD) hospital stay was 4.2±1.5 days in the drainage group, and 12.7±6.5 days in the surgery group (p<0.001). Over a mean follow-up period of 17 months, the mean cyst diameter decreased from 8.0±3.0 to 1.4±3.5 cm (p<0.001) after percutaneous drainage and from 9.1±3.0 to 0.9±1.8 cm (p<0.001) after surgery. The final cyst diameter did not differ significantly between the two groups (p=0.2). The cysts disappeared in 22 patients (88%) in the drainage group, and in 18 (72%) in the surgery group (p=0.29). After an initial rise, the echinococcal-antibody titers fell progressively, and at the last follow-up were negative (<1:160) in 19 patients (76%) in the drainage group, and 17 (68%) in the surgery group (p=0.74). There were procedure-related complications in 8 patients (32%) in the drainage group, and 21 (84%) in the surgery group, 17 of whom had fever postoperatively (p<0.001).

Conclusion

Percutaneous drainage, combined with albendazole therapy, is an effective and safe alternative to surgery for the treatment of uncomplicated hydatid cysts of the liver and requires a shorter hospital stay.

2. Pathogens

r. Enterococcal Infections

A Comparison of the Effect of Universal Use of Gloves and Gowns with That of Glove Use Alone on Acquisition of Vancomycin-Resistant Enterococci in a Medical Intensive Care Unit

Title	A comparison of the effect of universal use of gloves and gowns with that of glove use alone on acquisition of vancomycin-resistant enterococci in a medical intensive care unit.
Authors	Slaughter S, Hayden MK, Nathan C, et al.
Reference	Ann Intern Med 1996;125:448–456.
Disease/ Pathogen	Vancomycin resistant enterococci.
Purpose	To determine the efficacy of the use of gloves and gowns, compared with that of the use of gloves alone for the prevention of nosocomial transmission of vancomycin-resistant enterococci.
Design	Epidemiologic study and controlled, nonrandomized, clinical trial.
Patients	181 consecutive patients admitted to the medical intensive care unit for 48 hours or more.
Treatment/ prophylaxis regimen	It was determined that all hospital employees would always use gloves and gowns when attending eight particular beds in the medical intensive care unit and would always use gloves alone when attending eight others. Compliance with precautions was monitored weekly.

A Comparison of the Effect of Universal Use of Gloves and Gowns with That of Glove Use Alone on Acquisition of Vancomycin-Resistant Enterococci in a Medical Intensive Care Unit

(continued)

Results   The 93 patients in glove-and-gown rooms and the 88 patients in glove-only rooms had similar demographic and clinical characteristics. 15 (16.1%) patients in the glove-and-gown group, and 13 (14.8%) in the glove-only group had vancomycin-resistant enterococci on admission to the medical intensive care unit. 24 (25.8%) patients in the glove-and-gown group and 21 (23.9%) in the glove-only group acquired vancomycin-resistant enterococci in the medical intensive care unit. The mean times to colonization among the patients who became colonized were 8 days in the glove-and-gown group and 7.1 days in the glove-only group. None of these comparisons were statistically significant. Risk factors for acquisition of vancomycin-resistant enterococci included length of stay in the medical intensive care unit, use of enteral feeding, and use of sucralfate. Compliance with precautions was 79% in glove-and-gown rooms and 62% in glove-only rooms (p<0.001). Only 25 of 397 (6.3%) environmental cultures were positive for vancomycin-resistant enterococci. 19 types of vancomycin-resistant enterococci were documented by pulsed-field gel electrophoresis during the study period.

Conclusion   Universal use of gloves, and gowns was no better than universal use of gloves, only in preventing rectal colonization by vancomycin-resistant enterococci in a medical intensive care unit of a hospital in which vancomycin-resistant enterococci are endemic. Because the use of gowns and gloves together may be associated with better compliance, and may help prevent transmission of other infectious agents, this finding may not be applicable to outbreaks caused by single strains or hospitals in which the prevalence of vancomycin-resistant enterococci is low.

Title	Vancomycin-resistant Enterococcus faecium bacteremia: Risk factors for infection.
Authors	Edmond MB, Ober JF, Weinbaum DL, et al.
Reference	Clin Infect Dis 1995;20(5):1126–1133.
Disease/ Pathogen	Vancomycin-resistant E. faecium.
Purpose	To describe an outbreak of vancomycin-resistant E. faecium (vanA phenotype) bacteremia on the oncology ward of a tertiary care community hospital.
Design	Case control study.
Patients	11 cases with vancomycin-resistant E. faecium who received, on average, six antibiotic agents prior to the development of bacteremia, and 22 matched controls.

Vancomycin-Resistant Enterococcus Faecium Bacteremia: Risk Factors for Infection.

(continued)

Results

In 10 of the 11 cases, the patients had leukemia and were neutropenic (median duration of neutropenia, 21 days) at the time of bacteremia. On average, patients received six antibiotic agents, for a total of 61 agent-days prior to development of vancomycin-resistant E. faecium bacteremia. The mortality rate was 73%. Molecular typing of 22 isolates revealed that the majority (83%) represented a common strain, indicating nosocomial spread. When the 11 cases were compared to 22 matched control patients, gastrointestinal colonization with vancomycin-resistant E. faecium (odds ration [denominator, 0] infinity, p=0.005) and the use of antimicrobial agents with significant activity aginst anaerobes (metronidazole, clindamycin, and imipenem; odds ration infinity, p=0.02) were found to be risk factors for the development of vancomycin-resistant E. faecium bacteremia.

Conclusion

Since no proven therapy for such infection exists, there is an urgent need to identify effective measures to prevent and control the development of vancomycin-resistant E. faecium bacteremia.

2. Pathogens
s. Fungi

The Effect of Prophylactic Fluconazole on the Clinical Spectrum of Fungal Diseases in Bone Marrow Transplant Recipients with Special Attention to Hepatic Candidiasis: An Autopsy Study of 355 Patients.

Title	The effect of prophylactic fluconazole on the clinical spectrum of fungal diseases in bone marrow transplant recipients with special attention to hepatic candidiasis. An autopsy study of 355 patients.
Authors	van Burik JH, Leisenring W, Myerson D, et al.
Reference	Medicine 1998;77:246–254.
Disease/ Pathogen	Fungal infections.
Purpose	To determine whether fluconazole prophylaxis prevented visceral fungal infection.
Design	Autopsy review.
Patients	355 autopsies at a major marrow transplant center.
Treatment/ prophylaxis regimen	Fluconazole prophylaxis was defined by a minimum of 5 prophylactic doses.

The Effect of Prophylactic Fluconazole on the Clinical Spectrum of Fungal Diseases in Bone Marrow Transplant Recipients with Special Attention to Hepatic Candidiasis: An Autopsy Study of 355 Patients.

(continued)

Results

Fungal infection (any site) was found in 40% of patients transplanted and autopsied at the center. Overall, the proportion of autopsies with any fungal infection was not different for those patients receiving no fluconazole prophylaxis vs those with prophylactic fluconazole. With fluconazole prophylaxis, candidal infections were less frequent, decreasing from 27% to 8%, while Aspergillus infections were more frequent, increasing from 18% to 29%. No increase in deaths related to non-albicans Candida infections was seen. Of the 329 patients with livers examined, hepatic infection caused by Candida species was significantly less common in patients who had received fluconazole. Fungal liver infection was found in 31 patients (9%), 16% of those who were not treated with fluconazole and 3% of those who were treated with fluconazole. Since patients with candidal infections died earlier after marrow transplant than patients with mold infections, we speculate that a longer length of survival may dispose toward acquisition of mold infections.

Conclusion

Fluconazole prophylaxis in this cohort of marrow transplant patients undergoing autopsy resulted in a significant reduction in infection caused by Candida species and an increase in mold infections.

Effect of Prophylactic Fluconazole on the Frequency of Fungal Infections, Amphotericin B Use, and Health Care Costs in Patients Undergoing Intensive Chemotherapy for Hematologic Neoplasias

Title	Effect of prophylactic fluconazole on the frequency of fungal infections, amphotericin B use, and health care costs in patients undergoing intensive chemotherapy for hematologic neoplasias.
Authors	Schaffner A, Schaffner M.
Reference	J Infect Dis 1995;172(4):1035–1041.
Disease/ Pathogen	Fungal infections in patients with hematologic malignancy.
Purpose	To examine the effect of fluconazole therapy on the frequency of fungal infections, amphotericin B use, and health care costs in patients undergoing intensive chemotherapy for hematologic neoplasias.
Design	Double blind, controlled, single center trial.
Patients	96 consecutive patients undergoing 154 episodes of chemotherapy.
Follow-up	End points were amphotericin B use, fungal infection, stable neutrophil count >0.5 x 10(9)/L, toxicity precluding further fluconazole use, and death.
Treatment/ prophylaxis regimen	Patients received 400 mg of fluconazole or placebo until bone marrow recovery or initiation of intravenous amphotericin B infusions.

Effect of Prophylactic Fluconazole on the Frequency of Fungal Infections, Amphotericin B Use, and Health Care Costs in Patients Undergoing Intensive Chemotherapy for Hematologic Neoplasias

(continued)

Results
:   By Kaplan-Meier estimation, the time to initiation of amphotericin B therapy was shorter in 76 patients treated with placebo than in 75 treated with fluconazole (p=0.003). Also, fluconazole reduced the number of febrile days by 20% (p=0.002) and prevented oropharyngeal candidiasis (1/75 vs 9/76, p=0.018). The frequency of deep mycoses (8/76 vs 8/75) and outcome were unaffected.

Conclusion
:   Fluconazole did not have a favorable effect on infection-related health care costs and was associated with prolonged severe neutropenia (p=0.01).

2. Pathogens
t. Gonorrhea

A Comparison of Single-Dose Cefixime with Ceftriaxone as Treatment for Uncomplicated Gonorrhea

Title	A comparison of single-dose cefixime with ceftriaxone as treatment for uncomplicated gonorrhea.
Authors	Handsfield HH, McCormack WM, Hook EW 3d, et al.
Reference	New Engl J Med 1991;325:1337–1341.
Disease/ Pathogen	Gonorrhea.
Purpose	To compare single-dose cefixime with ceftriaxone as a treatment for uncomplicated gonorrhea.
Design	Randomized, unblinded, multicenter study.
Patients	209 men and 124 women with uncomplicated gonorrhea.
Treatment/ prophylaxis regimen	Three single-dose treatment regimens: 400 mg or 800 mg of cefixime, administered orally, or 250 mg of ceftriaxone administered intramuscularly.

A Comparison of Single-Dose Cefixime with Ceftriaxone as Treatment for Uncomplicated Gonorrhea

Results   The overall cure rates were 96% for the 400 mg dose of cefixime (89 of 93 patients) (95% confidence interval [CI] 93.5%–97.8%); 98% for the 800 mg dose of cefixime (86 of 88 patients) (95% CI 94.6%–100%); and 98% for ceftriaxone (92 of 94 patients) (95% CI 94.9%–100%). The cure rates were similar in men and women, and pharyngeal infection was eradicated in 20 of 22 patients (91%). 39% of 303 pre-treatment gonococcal isolates had one or more types of antimicrobial resistance; the efficacy of all three regimens was independent of the resistance pattern. Chlamydia trachomatis infection persisted in at least half the patients infected in each treatment group. All three regimens were well tolerated.

Conclusion   In the treatment of uncomplicated gonorrhea, a single dose of cefixime (400 or 800 mg) given orally appears to be as effective as the currently recommended regimen of ceftriaxone (250 mg given intramuscularly).

2. Pathogens

u. Helicobacter Pylori Infection

Title	Randomised trial of eradication of Helicobacter pylori before non-steroidal anti-inflammatory drug therapy to prevent peptic ulcers.
Authors	Chan FK, Sung JJ, Chung SC, et al.
Reference	Lancet 1997;350:975–979.
Disease/ Pathogen	Helicobacter pylori.
Purpose	To study the efficacy of eradication of H. pylori in the prevention of NSAID-induced peptic ulcers.
Design	Randomized, controlled trial.
Patients	Patients with musculoskeletal pain who required NSAID treatment. None of the patients had previous exposure to NSAID therapy.
Follow-up	Endoscopy was repeated after 8 weeks of naproxen treatment or when naproxen treatment was stopped early because of bleeding or intractable dyspepsia. All endoscopic examinations were done by one endoscopist who was unaware of treatment assignment. The primary end point was the cumulative rate of gastric and duodenal ulcers.
Treatment/ prophylaxis regimen	Patients who had H. pylori infection but no pre-existing ulcers on endoscopy were randomly allocated naproxen alone (750 mg daily) for 8 weeks or a 1-week course of triple therapy (bismuth subcitrate 120 mg, tetracycline 500 mg, metronidazole 400 mg, each given orally four times daily) before administration of naproxen (750 mg daily).

(continued)

Results

202 patients underwent endoscopic screening for enrollment in the trial, and 100 eligible patients were randomly assigned treatment. 92 patients completed the trial (47
in the naproxen group, 45 in the triple-therapy group). At
8 weeks, H. pylori had been eradicated from no patients
in the naproxen group and 40 (89%) in the triple-therapy
group (p<0.001). 12 (26%) naproxen-group patients
developed ulcers: Five had ulcer pain and one developed
ulcer bleeding. Only three (7%) patients on triple therapy had ulcers, and two of these patients had failure of H.
pylori eradication (p=0.01). Thus, 12 (26%) patients with
persistent H. pylori infection but only one (3%) with successful H. pylori eradication developed ulcers with
naproxen (p=0.002).

Conclusion

Eradication of H. pylori before NSAID therapy reduces the
occurrence of NSAID-induced peptic ulcers.

Lack of Effect of Treating Helicobacter Pylori Infection in Patients with Nonulcer Dyspepsia

Title	Lack of effect of treating Helicobacter pylori infection in patients with nonulcer dyspepsia.
Authors	Blum AL, Talley NJ, O'Morain C, et al.
Reference	N Engl J Med 1998;339:1875–1881.
Disease/ Pathogen	Nonulcer dyspepsia.
Purpose	To compare the effect of 1 week of treatment with omeprazole, amoxicillin, and clarithromycin with that of 1 week of treatment with omeprazole alone on the relief of symptoms, eradication of H. pylori infection, healing of gastritis, and quality of life in patients with nonulcer dyspepsia.
Design	Randomized, double blind, multicenter.
Patients	348 patients were randomly assigned to a treatment group.
Follow-up	1 year.
Treatment/ prophylaxis regimen	20 mg of omeprazole twice daily (morning and evening), 1000 mg of amoxicillin twice daily, and 500 mg of clarithromycin twice daily or 20 mg of omeprazole twice daily, as well as placebo antibiotics.

Lack of Effect of Treating Helicobacter Pylori Infection in Patients with Nonulcer Dyspepsia

(continued)

Results	20 of the 348 patients were excluded after randomization because they were not infected with H. pylori, were not treated, or had no data available. For the remaining 328 patients (164 in each group), treatment was successful for 27.4% of those assigned to receive omeprazole and antibiotics and 20.7% of those assigned to receive omeprazole alone (p=0.17; absolute difference between groups 6.7%; 95% confidence interval [CI] -2.6–16). After 12 months, gastritis had healed in 75% of the patients in the group given omeprazole and antibiotics and in 3% of the patients in the omeprazole group (p<0.001); the respective rates of H. pylori eradication were 79% and 2%. In the group given omeprazole and antibiotics, the rate of treatment success among patients with persistent H. pylori infection was similar to that among patients in whom the infection was eradicated (26% vs 31%). There were no significant differences between the groups in the quality of life after treatment.
Conclusion	In patients with nonulcer dyspepsia, the eradication of H. pylori infection is not likely to relieve symptoms.

Disappearance of Hyperplastic Polyps in the Stomach after Eradication of Helicobacter Pylori: A Randomized, Controlled Trial.

Title	Disappearance of hyperplastic polyps in the stomach after eradication of Helicobacter pylori: A randomized, controlled trial.
Authors	Ohkusa T, Takashimizu I, Fujiki K, et al.
Reference	Ann Intern Med 1998;129:712–715.
Disease/ Pathogen	Helicobacter pylori infection.
Purpose	To determine if hyperplastic polyps would disappear after eradication of H. pylori.
Design	Randomized, controlled trial.
Patients	35 patients (19 men and 16 women; age range 29–75 years) with H. pylori infection and hyperplastic polyps of the stomach diagnosed by endoscopic biopsy.
Follow-up	3–15 months (average, 7.1±1.2 months).
Treatment/ prophylaxis regimen	In the treatment group a proton-pump inhibitor (omeprazole or lansoprazole), amoxicillin, and either clarithromycin or ecabet sodium; in the control group (n=18), patients had endoscopic examination but did not receive treatment.

Disappearance of Hyperplastic Polyps in the Stomach after Eradication of Helicobacter Pylori: A Randomized, Controlled Trial.

(continued)

Results	In the treatment group, the polyps had disappeared by 3-15 months (average 7.1±1.2 months) after the end of treatment in 12 of all 17 patients (71%) and in 12 of the 15 patients (80%) in whom H. pylori was eradicated. However, 12-15 months after the start of the study, no change in polyps or H. pylori status was seen in any controls (p<0.001). Histologic findings of inflammation and activity, serum gastrin levels, and titers of IgG to H. pylori showed significant regression in the treatment group, compared with the control group (p<0.01).
Conclusion	Most hyperplastic polyps disappeared after eradication of H. pylori. Thus, eradication should be attempted before endoscopic removal is done in patients with hyperplastic gastric polyps and H. pylori infection.

Effect of Treatment of Helicobacter Pylori Infection on the Long-Term Recurrence of Gastric or Duodenal Ulcer: A Randomized, Controlled Study.

Title	Effect of treatment of Helicobacter pylori infection on the long-term recurrence of gastric or duodenal ulcer: A randomized, controlled study.
Authors	Graham DY, Lew GM, Klein PD, et al.
Reference	Ann Intern Med 1992;116:705–708.
Disease/ Pathogen	Helicobacter pylori.
Purpose	To determine the effect of treating H. pylori infection on the recurrence of gastric and duodenal ulcer disease.
Design	Follow-up of up to 2 years in patients with healed ulcers who had participated in randomized, controlled trials.
Patients	A total of 109 patients infected with H. pylori who had a recently healed duodenal (83 patients) or gastric ulcer (26 patients) as confirmed by endoscopy.
Follow-up	Endoscopy to assess ulcer recurrence was done at 3-month intervals, or when a patient developed symptoms, for a maximum of 2 years.

Effect of Treatment of Helicobacter Pylori Infection on the Long-Term Recurrence of Gastric or Duodenal Ulcer: A Randomized, Controlled Study.

(continued)

Treatment/ prophylaxis regimen	Patients received ranitidine, 300 mg, or ranitidine plus triple therapy. Triple therapy consisted of tetracycline, 2 g; metronidazole, 750 mg; and bismuth subsalicylate, 5 or 8 tablets (151 mg bismuth per tablet), and was administered for the first 2 weeks of treatment; ranitidine therapy was continued until the ulcer had healed or 16 weeks had elapsed. After ulcer healing, no maintenance anti-ulcer therapy was given.
Results	The probability of recurrence for patients who received triple therapy plus ranitidine was significantly lower than that for patients who received ranitidine alone: For patients with duodenal ulcer, 12% (95% confidence interval [CI] 1%–24%) compared with 95% (CI 84%–100%); for patients with gastric ulcer, 13% (CI 4%–31%), compared with 74% (44%–100%). Fifty percent of patients who received ranitidine alone for healing of duodenal or gastric ulcer had a relapse within 12 weeks of healing. Ulcer recurrence in the triple therapy group was related to the failure to eradicate H. pylori and to the use of nonsteroidal anti-inflammatory drugs.
Conclusion	Eradication of H. pylori infection markedly changes the natural history of peptic ulcer in patients with duodenal or gastric ulcer. Most peptic ulcers associated with H. pylori infection are curable.

Effect of Triple Therapy (Antibiotics Plus Bismuth) on Duodenal Ulcer Healing: A Randomized, Controlled Trial.

Title	Effect of triple therapy (antibiotics plus bismuth) on duodenal ulcer healing: A randomized, controlled trial.
Authors	Graham DY, Lew GM, Evans DG, et al.
Reference	Ann of Intern Med 1991;115:266–269.
Disease/Pathogen	Duodenal ulcer.
Purpose	To determine whether antimicrobial therapy for Helicobacter pylori infection accelerates the healing of duodenal ulcers.
Design	Single blind, randomized, controlled trial.
Patients	105 patients with endoscopically verified duodenal ulcers.
Follow-up	Videoendoscopic assessment of ulcer status was done until ulcer healing was complete. Evaluations were done after 2, 4, 8, 12, and 16 weeks of therapy.
Treatment/prophylaxis regimen	Patients received either ranitidine, 300 mg/d, or ranitidine, 300 mg/d, plus "triple therapy" (2 g/d of tetracycline, 750 mg/d of metronidazole, and 5 or 8 bismuth subsalicylate tablets per day). Triple therapy was administered for only the first 2 weeks of ulcer treatment.

Results   Ulcer healing was more rapid in patients receiving raniti-
               dine plus triple therapy than in patients receiving raniti-
               dine alone (p<0.01). The cumulative percentages of
               patients with healed ulcers in the group receiving raniti-
               dine plus triple therapy and in the group receiving raniti-
               dine alone were as follows: 37% and 18% after week 2;
               74% and 53% after week 4; 84% and 68% after week 8;
               96% and 80% after week 12; and 98% and 84% after week
               16.

Conclusion   Combined therapy with anti-H. pylori agents and raniti-
               dine was superior to ranitidine alone for duodenal ulcer
               healing.

2. Pathogens

v. Herpes Simplex Virus Infections

Use of Brain Biopsy for Diagnostic Evaluation of Patients with Suspected Herpes Simplex Encephalitis: A Statistical Model and Its Clinical Implications.

Title	Use of brain biopsy for diagnostic evaluation of patients with suspected herpes simplex encephalitis: A statistical model and its clinical implications.
Authors	Soong SJ, Watson NE, Caddell GR, et al.
Reference	J Infect Dis 1991;163(1):17–22.
Disease/ Pathogen	Herpes simplex encephalitis (HSE).
Purpose	To define the utility of brain biopsy for diagnostic evaluation of patients with suspected HSE.
Treatment/ prophylaxis regimen	Two strategies were compared: Strategy I, brain biopsy with acyclovir (ACV) treatment for 10 days in biopsy-positive patients, and strategy II, ACV therapy without brain biopsy.
Results	Strategy I resulted in a greater 6-month survival rate when the likelihood of patients having HSE was less than 70%. Based on the current estimated prevalence of HSE (for patients with suspected HSE) of 35%, strategy I showed a slight advantage of a 3.2% increase in 6-month survival rate. An individual patient's chance of a positive brain biopsy can be predicted using a mathematical equation based on several important clinical assessments.
Conclusion	This equation, in conjunction with the decision analysis, is a useful guide for the clinical management of patients with regard to brain biopsy.

Acyclovir for the Prevention of Recurrent Herpes Simplex Virus Eye Disease

Title	Acyclovir for the prevention of recurrent herpes simplex virus eye disease.
Authors	The Herpetic Eye Disease Study Group.
Reference	N Engl J Med 1998;339:300–306.
Disease/ Pathogen	Herpes simplex virus (HSV) eye disease.
Purpose	To determine whether treatment with 400 mg of oral acyclovir twice daily for 1 year would prevent ocular recurrences in immunocompetent persons who had had an episode of ocular HSV within the preceding year.
Design	Randomized, double blind, placebo controlled, multicenter.
Patients	703 immunocompetent patients who had had ocular HSV disease.
Follow-up	12 month-treatment period and 6 month observation period.
Treatment/ prophylaxis regimen	400 mg of acyclovir orally twice daily for 12 months or two placebo capsules twice daily.

Results   The cumulative probability of a recurrence of any type of ocular HSV disease during the 12-month treatment period was 19% in the acyclovir group and 32% in the placebo group (p<0.001). Among the 337 patients with a history of stromal keratitis, the most common serious form of ocular HSV disease, the cumulative probability of recurrent stromal keratitis was 14% in the acyclovir group and 28% in the placebo group (p=0.005). The cumulative probability of a recurrence of nonocular (primarily orofacial) HSV disease was also lower in the acyclovir group than in the placebo group (19% vs 36%, p<0.001). There was no rebound in the rate of HSV disease in the six months after treatment with acyclovir was stopped.

Conclusion   After the resolution of ocular HSV disease, 12 months of treatment with acyclovir reduces the rate of recurrent ocular HSV disease and orofacial HSV disease. Long-term antiviral prophylaxis is most important for patients with a history of HSV stromal keratitis, since it can prevent additional episodes and potential loss of vision.

Oral Famciclovir for the Suppression of Recurrent Genital Herpes: A Randomized, Controlled Trial.

Title	Oral famciclovir for the suppression of recurrent genital herpes: A randomized, controlled trial.
Authors	Diaz-Mitoma F, Sibbald RG, Shafran SD, et al.
Reference	JAMA 1998;280:887–892.
Disease/ Pathogen	Gential herpes.
Purpose	To determine the efficacy and safety of famciclovir in the suppression of recurrent genital herpes simplex virus (HSV) infection.
Design	A randomized, double blind, placebo controlled, multi-center, parallel group study.
Patients	A total of 455 patients (223 men, 232 women) aged 18 years or older with a history of 6 or more episodes of genital herpes during 12 of the most recent 24 months, in the absence of suppressive therapy, received study medication.
Follow-up	Time to the first recurrence of genital HSV infection; the proportion of patients remaining free of HSV recurrence at 6 months; frequency of adverse events.
Treatment/ prophylaxis regimen	Oral famciclovir, 125 mg or 250 mg, 3 times daily or 250 mg twice daily, or placebo for 52 weeks.

Oral Famciclovir for the Suppression of Recurrent Genital Herpes: A Randomized, Controlled Trial.

(continued)

Results   In an intent-to-treat analysis, famciclovir significantly delayed the time to the first recurrence of genital herpes at all dose regimens (hazard ratio 2.9–3.3; p<.001); median time to recurrence for famciclovir recipients was 222–336 days, compared with 47 days for placebo recipients. The proportion of patients remaining free of HSV recurrence was approximately 3 times higher in famciclovir recipients (79%–86%) than in placebo recipients (27%) at 6 months (relative risk 2.9–3.1; p<.001); efficacy was maintained at 12 months. Famciclovir was well tolerated with an adverse experience profile comparable to placebo.

Conclusion   Oral famciclovir (125 mg or 250 mg 3 times daily, or 250 mg twice daily) is an effective, well tolerated treatment for the suppression of genital HSV infection in patients with frequent recurrences.

Title	Suppression of subclinical shedding of herpes simplex virus type 2 with acyclovir.
Authors	Wald A, Zeh J, Barnum GA, et al.
Reference	Ann Intern Med 1996;124:8–15.
Disease/ Pathogen	Herpes simplex virus type 2 (HSV-2).
Purpose	To assess the effect of the antiviral drug acyclovir on the frequency of subclinical shedding of herpes simplex virus (HSV) in the genital tract.
Design	A double blind, placebo controlled, crossover, clinical trial.
Patients	34 women with herpes simplex virus type 2 (HSV-2) antibody only, and genital herpes of less than 2 years' duration.
Follow-up	140 days.
Treatment/ prophylaxis regimen	Participants were randomly assigned to receive either acyclovir, 400 mg twice daily for 70 days, followed by a 14-day washout period, and then placebo for 70 days, or the study medications in the reverse order.

Results   In an intent-to-treat analysis of the initial treatment period, 15 of the 17 women who received placebo and three of the 17 women who received acyclovir had at least 1 day of subclinical shedding (p<0.001). Among the participants who received placebo, subclinical shedding occurred on 64 of 928 (6.9%) days compared with 3 of 1057 (0.3%) days among the participants who received acyclovir (p<0.001). The relative risk for subclinical shedding was 0.09 (95% confidence interval [CI] 0.03–0.35) for the women who received acyclovir, compared with the women who received placebo. In a paired analysis of 26 women who completed both arms of the study, acyclovir therapy was associated with a decrease in the frequency of subclinical shedding; subclinical shedding occurred on 83 of 1439 (5.8%) days with placebo, and on 6 of 1611 (0.37%) days with acyclovir (p<0.001)—a 94% reduction. The frequency of subclinical shedding was reduced at all anatomic sites and in all patients.

Conclusion   Daily therapy with oral acyclovir suppresses subclinical shedding of HSV-2 in the genital tract, suggesting that studies to evaluate the use of acyclovir in preventing HSV-2 transmission are warranted.

Famciclovir for the Treatment of Acute Herpes Zoster: Effects on Acute Disease and Postherpetic Neuralgia: A Randomized, Double Blind, Placebo Controlled Trial.

Title	Famciclovir for the treatment of acute herpes zoster: Effects on acute disease and postherpetic neuralgia: A randomized, double blind, placebo controlled trial.
Authors	Tyring S, Barbarash RA, Nahlik JE, et al.
Reference	Ann Intern Med 1995;123:89–96.
Disease/ Pathogen	Herpes zoster.
Purpose	To document the effects of treatment with famciclovir on the acute signs and symptoms of herpes zoster and postherpetic neuralgia.
Design	A randomized, double blind, placebo controlled, multicenter trial.
Patients	419 immunocompetent adults with uncomplicated herpes zoster.
Follow-up	5 months.
Treatment/ prophylaxis regimen	Patients were assigned within 72 hours of rash onset to famciclovir, 500 mg; famciclovir, 750 mg; or placebo, three times daily for 7 days.

Famciclovir for the Treatment of Acute Herpes Zoster: Effects on Acute Disease and Postherpetic Neuralgia: A Randomized, Double Blind, Placebo Controlled Trial.

(continued)

Results
Famciclovir was well tolerated, with a safety profile similar to that of placebo. Famciclovir accelerated lesion healing and reduced the duration of viral shedding. Most importantly, famciclovir recipients had faster resolution of postherpetic neuralgia (approximately twofold faster) than placebo recipients; differences between the placebo group and both the 500-mg famciclovir group (hazard ratio 1.7 [95% confidence interval (CI) 1.1–2.7]) and the 750-mg famciclovir group (hazard ratio 1.9 [CI, 1.2–2.9]) were statistically significant (p=0.02 and 0.01, respectively). The median duration of postherpetic neuralgia was reduced by approximately 2 months.

Conclusion
Oral famciclovir, 500 mg or 750 mg three times daily for 7 days, is an effective and well tolerated therapy for herpes zoster that decreases the duration of the disease's most debilitating complication, postherpetic neuralgia.

Oral Acyclovir to Suppress Frequently Recurrent Herpes Labialis: A Double Blind, Placebo Controlled Trial.

Title	Oral acyclovir to suppress frequently recurrent herpes labialis: A double blind, placebo controlled trial.
Authors	Rooney JF, Straus SE, Mannix ML, et al.
Reference	Ann Intern Med 1993;118:268–272.
Disease/ Pathogen	Herpes labialis.
Purpose	To determine whether oral acyclovir reduces the incidence of recurrent herpes labialis in otherwise healthy patients with proven frequently recurrent disease.
Design	Randomized, double blind, placebo controlled, crossover trial.
Patients	56 otherwise healthy adults who reported frequently recurrent herpes labialis (≥6 episodes/per year) were enrolled into the study. During a 4-month observation period, 22 patients had herpes labialis two or more times, and were eligible for study treatment.
Follow-up	Recurrent outbreaks were determined by examination and by viral culture.
Treatment/ prophylaxis regimen	22 patients were randomized to receive either acyclovir, 400 mg twice daily, or matched placebo for 4 months. After the first treatment period, patients were given the alternate treatment for another 4 months and were then taken off study medication to observe the first post-treatment recurrence.

Results   20 patients completed blind treatment with both acyclovir and placebo. The median time to first clinically documented recurrence was 46 days for placebo courses and 118 days for acyclovir courses (p=0.05). The mean number of recurrences per 4-month treatment period was 1.8 episodes per patient during placebo treatment, and 0.85 episodes per patient during acyclovir treatment (p=0.009). The mean number of virologically confirmed recurrences per patient was 1.4 with placebo therapy, compared with 0.4 with acyclovir (p=0.003).

Conclusion   Oral acyclovir, 400 mg twice daily, is effective in suppressing herpes labialis in immunocompetent adults confirmed to have frequently recurrent infection. Treatment with acyclovir in this study resulted in a 53% reduction in the number of clinical recurrences and a 71% reduction in virus culture-positive recurrences compared with placebo therapy.

2. Pathogens

w. Herpes Simplex/Herpes Zoster Virus Infections

Comparison of Tzanck Smear, Viral Culture, and
DNA Diagnostic Methods in Detection of Herpes Simplex and
Varicella-Zoster Infection

Title	Comparison of Tzanck smear, viral culture, and DNA diagnostic methods in detection of herpes simplex and varicella-zoster infection.
Authors	Nahass GT, Goldstein BA, Zhu WY, et al.
Reference	JAMA 1992;268:2541–2544.
Disease/ Pathogen	Herpes.
Purpose	To compare Tzanck smears, viral cultures, and DNA diagnostic methods using the polymerase chain reaction (PCR) in detection of herpes simplex virus (HSV) or varicella-zoster virus (VZV) infection in clinically suspected cases.
Design	A 12-month trial comparing PCR with viral cultures and Tzanck smears in patients with clinically suspected HSV or VZV infection.
Patients	Convenience samples of patients clinically suspected to have HSV (n=48) or VZV (n=35). To be included in the final analysis, patients needed to have a positive Tzanck smear, viral culture, or PCR result. Patients who were clinically suspected to have HSV but had VZV by viral culture or PCR, were analyzed in the VZV group. Similarly, patients who were clinically suspected to have VZV, but had HSV by viral culture or PCR, were analyzed in the HSV group. 77 patients were available for final analysis: HSV (n=30), VZV (n=32), and 15 control cases who did not have evidence of viral infection.

Comparison of Tzanck Smear, Viral Culture, and DNA Diagnostic Methods in Detection of Herpes Simplex and Varicella-Zoster Infection

(continued)

Results	For HSV, PCR detected HSV DNA sequences in 73% of stained smears and 83% of unstained smears. For VZV infection, VZV DNA sequences were detected in 88% of stained smears and 97% of unstained smears. Viral DNA sequences were not detected in the 15 control cases. Viral cultures were positive in 83% and 44% of HSV and VZV cases, respectively. The Tzanck smear was positive in 60% and 75% of HSV and VZV cases, respectively.
Conclusion	PCR is a reliable method for detecting HSV and VZV DNA sequences from single stained and unstained Tzanck smears. It is clearly superior to viral culture in identifying VZV infection and is equivalent to conventional culture techniques in identifying cases of HSV.

Disseminated Herpes Zoster in the Immunocompromised Host in a Comparative Trial of Acyclovir and Vidarabine: The NIAID Collaborative Antiviral Study Group.

Title	Disseminated herpes zoster in the immunocompromised host in a comparative trial of acyclovir and vidarabine: The NIAID Collaborative Antiviral Study Group.
Authors	Whitley RJ, Gnann JW Jr., Hinthorn D, et al.
Reference	J Infect Dis 1992;165(3):450–455.
Disease/ Pathogen	Herpes zoster.
Design	Double blind, controlled trial.
Patients	73 immunocompromised patients with disseminated herpes zoster.
Treatment/ prophylaxis regimen	Acyclovir (n=37) was administered at 30 mg/kg/day at 8-hour intervals and vidarabine (n=36) was given as a continuous 12-hour infusion at 10 mg/kg/day for 7 days (longer if resolution of cutaneous or visceral disease was incomplete).
Results	No demographic differences existed between treatment groups. No deaths attributable to varicella-zoster virus infection occurred within 1 month of treatment. Neither rates of cutaneous healing, resolution of acute neuritis, and frequency of postherpetic neuralgia nor adverse clinical and laboratory events differed between treatment groups. Acyclovir recipients were discharged from the hospital more promptly than vidarabine recipients (p=0.04, log rank test).
Conclusion	These data indicate that disseminated herpes zoster is amenable to therapy with either acyclovir or vidarabine; resultant mortality is low.

Treatment of Adult Varicella with Oral Acyclovir: A Randomized, Placebo Controlled Trial.

Title	Treatment of adult varicella with oral acyclovir: A randomized, placebo controlled trial.
Authors	Wallace MR, Bowler WA, Murray NB, et al.
Reference	Ann Intern Med 1992;117:358–363.
Disease/ Pathogen	Varicella.
Purpose	To assess the efficacy of oral acyclovir in treating adults with varicella and to describe the natural history of adult varicella.
Design	Double blind, placebo controlled, randomized trial.
Patients	148 of 206 consecutive adult active duty Navy and Marine Corps personnel, who were hospitalized for isolation and inpatient therapy of varicella and, who could be treated within 72 hours of rash onset completed the study. The diagnosis of varicella was confirmed by acute and convalescent serology in 143 of 144 patients with available paired sera.
Follow-up	Daily lesion counts, symptom scores, temperature measurements, and laboratory tests were used to monitor the course of the illness.
Treatment/ prophylaxis regimen	Patients were randomly assigned to receive either acyclovir, 800 mg orally five times per day for 7 days, or an identical placebo. Separate randomization codes were used for patients presenting within 24 hours of rash onset and for those presenting 25–72 hours after rash onset.

(continued)

Results   Early treatment (initiated within 24 hours of rash onset) reduced the total time to (100%) crusting, from 7.4 to 5.6 days (p=0.001) and reduced the maximum number of lesions by 46% (p=0.04). Duration of fever and severity of symptoms were also reduced by early therapy. Late therapy (25–72 hours after rash onset) had no effect on the course of illness. Only four patients had pneumonia, and no encephalitis or mortality was noted.

Conclusion   Early therapy with oral acyclovir decreases the time to cutaneous healing of adult varicella, decreases the duration of fever, and lessens symptoms. Initiation of therapy after the first day of illness is of no value in uncomplicated cases of adult varicella. The low frequency of serious complications of varicella (pneumonia, encephalitis, or death) precluded any evaluation of the possible effect of acyclovir on these outcomes.

A Controlled Trial of Acyclovir for Chickenpox in Normal Children

Title	A controlled trial of acyclovir for chickenpox in normal children.
Authors	Dunkle LM, Arvin AM, Whitley RJ, et al.
Reference	New Engl J Med 1991;325:1539–1544.
Disease/ Pathogen	Chickenpox.
Purpose	To evaluate the effectiveness of acyclovir for the treatment of chickenpox.
Design	Multicenter, double blind, placebo controlled study
Patients	815 healthy children 2–12 years old who contracted chickenpox.
Treatment/ prophylaxis regimen	Treatment with acyclovir was begun within the first 24 hours of rash, and was administered by the oral route in a dose of 20 mg per kilogram of body weight four times daily for 5 days.

A Controlled Trial of Acyclovir for Chickenpox in Normal Children

(continued)

Results   The children treated with acyclovir had fewer varicella lesions than those given placebo (mean number, 294 vs 347; p<0.001), and a smaller proportion of them had more than 500 lesions (21%, as compared with 3% with placebo; p<0.001). In over 95% of the recipients of acyclovir, no new lesions formed after day 3, whereas new lesions were forming in 20% of the placebo recipients on day 6 or later. The recipients of acyclovir also had accelerated progression to the crusted and healed stages, less itching, and fewer residual lesions after 28 days. In the children treated with acyclovir, the duration of fever and constitutional symptoms was limited to 3–4 days, whereas in 20% of the children given placebo, illness lasted more than 4 days. There was no significant difference between groups in the distribution of 11 disease complications (10 bacterial skin infections and 1 case of transient cerebellar ataxia). Acyclovir was well tolerated, and there was no significant difference between groups in the titers of antibodies against varicella-zoster virus.

Conclusion   Acyclovir is a safe treatment that reduces the duration and severity of chickenpox in normal children when therapy is initiated during the first 24 hours of rash. Whether treatment with acyclovir can reduce the rare, serious complications of chickenpox remains uncertain.

2. Pathogens

x. Herpes Zoster Infections

Title	Herpes zoster: Risk categories for persistent pain.
Authors	Whitley RJ, Weiss HL, Soong SJ, et al.
Reference	J Infect Dis 1999;179(1):9-15.
Disease/ Pathogen	Herpes-zoster.
Purpose	To evaluate acute neuritis and persistent pain as measures to initiate clinical therapy.
Patients	Patients with herpes zoster categorized according to pain severity and number of lesions at presentation.
Follow-up	Risk categories were defined according to the magnitude of risk ratios (RRs) and a comparison of Kaplan-Meier survival estimates. For acute neuritis and zoster-associated pain, RRs defined rate of resolution.
Results	Patients who presented with severe or incapacitating pain, and a large number of lesions, were less likely to achieve resolution of both acute neuritis and zoster-associated pain (RR 18; 95% confidence interval [CI] 6.6-48.6, and RR 5.3; 95% CI 4.2-17.2, respectively).
Conclusion	These analyses identify the subgroups of patients for whom aggressive interventions are most strongly indicated.

Postherpetic Neuralgia: Impact of Famciclovir, Age, Rash Severity, and Acute Pain in Herpes Zoster Patients.

Title	Postherpetic neuralgia: Impact of famciclovir, age, rash severity, and acute pain in herpes zoster patients.
Authors	Dworkin RH, Boon RJ, Griffin DR, et al.
Reference	J Infect Dis 1998;178 Suppl 1:S76-80.
Disease/ Pathogen	Herpes.
Purpose	To examine the effect of famciclovir treatment on the duration of postherpetic neuralgia (PHN).
Design	Placebo controlled trial.
Patients	Patients with pain persisting after rash healing, pain persisting >30 days after study enrollment, or pain persisting >3 months after study enrollment.
Follow-up	30–180 days post-enrollment
Treatment/ prophylaxis regimen	Patients were assigned to receive either famciclovir or placebo.
Results	The results of these analyses indicated that greater age, rash severity, and acute pain severity are risk factors for prolonged PHN. In addition, they demonstrated that treatment of acute herpes zoster patients with famciclovir significantly reduces both the duration and prevalence of PHN.
Conclusion	Treatment of herpes zoster with famciclovir is effective.

2. Pathogens

y. Histoplasmosis

Title	Fluconazole therapy for histoplasmosis.
Authors	McKinsey DS, Kauffman CA, Pappas PG, et al.
Reference	Clin Infect Dis. 23(5):996–1001, 1996 Nov.
Disease/ Pathogen	Histoplasmosis.
Purpose	To assess the efficacy of oral fluconazole (200-800 mg daily) in the treatment of non-life-threatening acute pulmonary histoplasmosis, chronic pulmonary histoplasmosis, or disseminated histoplasmosis in patients without human immunodeficiency virus infection.
Design	Prospective trial.
Patients	Of 27 evaluable patients, two had progressive acute pulmonary histoplasmosis, 11 had chronic pulmonary histoplasmosis, and 14 had disseminated histoplasmosis.
Follow-up	Median durations of treatment in each of the three groups were 6 months, 7 months, and 11 months, respectively.
Treatment/ prophylaxis regimen	19 patients were treated with 400 mg of fluconazole daily (two of these patients received 800 mg daily for a portion of their treatment courses), seven were treated with 200 mg daily, and one was treated with 800 mg daily.

Results	Treatment was successful in 17 (63%) of 27 cases. Both of the patients with acute pulmonary infection responded to therapy, as did five (46%) of 11 patients with chronic pulmonary infection and 10 (71%) of 14 patients with disseminated infection. No substantial toxicity was observed.
Conclusion	The authors conclude that fluconazole therapy for histoplasmosis is only moderately effective, and should be reserved for patients who cannot take itraconazole.

2. Pathogens

z. Infectious Mononucleosis

Acyclovir and Prednisolone Treatment of Acute Infectious Mononucleosis: A Multicenter, Double Blind, Placebo Controlled Study.

Title	Acyclovir and prednisolone treatment of acute infectious mononucleosis: A multicenter, double blind, placebo controlled study.
Authors	Tynell E, Aurelius E, Brandell A, et al.
Reference	J Infect Dis 1996;174(2):324-331.
Disease/ Pathogen	Infectious mononucleosis.
Purpose	To evaluate the efficacy of acyclovir and prednisolone for the treatment of infectious mononucleosis.
Design	Multicenter, double blind, placebo controlled study.
Patients	94 patients with infectious mononucleosis and symptoms ≤7 days.
Treatment/ prophylaxis regimen	Patients were randomized to treatment with oral acyclovir (800 mg 5 times/day) and prednisolone (0.7 mg/kg for the first 4 days, which was reduced by 0.1 mg/kg on consecutive days for another 6 days; n=48), or placebo (n=46) for 10 days.

Acyclovir and Prednisolone Treatment of Acute Infectious Mononucleosis: A Multicenter, Double Blind, Placebo Controlled Study.

(continued)

Results

Oropharyngeal Epstein-Barr virus (EBV) shedding was significantly inhibited during the treatment period (p=0.02, Mann-Whitney rank test). No significant effect was observed for duration of general illness, sore throat, weight loss, or absence from school or work. The frequency of latent EBV-infected B lymphocytes in peripheral blood and the HLA-restricted EBV-specific cellular immunity, measured 6 months after onset of disease, was not affected by treatment.

Conclusion

Acyclovir combined with prednisolone inhibited oropharyngeal EBV replication without affecting duration of clinical symptoms or development of EBV-specific cellular immunity.

2. Pathogens

aa. Influenza

The Efficacy of Influenza Vaccination in Elderly Individuals:
A Randomized, Double Blind, Placebo Controlled Trial.

Title	The efficacy of influenza vaccination in elderly individuals: A randomized, double blind, placebo controlled trial.
Authors	Govaert TM, Thijs CT, Masurel N, et al.
Reference	JAMA 1994;272:1661–1665.
Disease/ Pathogen	Influenza.
Purpose	To determine the efficacy of influenza vaccination in elderly people.
Design	Randomized, double blind, placebo controlled trial, multi-center.
Patients	A total of 1838 subjects aged 60 years or older, not known as belonging to those high-risk groups in which vaccination was previously given.
Follow-up	Patients presenting with influenza-like illness, up to 5 months after vaccination; self-reported influenza in postal questionnaires 10 weeks and 5 months after vaccination; serological influenza (fourfold increase of antibody titer between 3 weeks and 5 months after vaccination).
Treatment/ prophylaxis regimen	Purified split-virion vaccine containing A/Singapore/ 6/86(H1N1), A/Beijing/353/89(H3N2), B/Beijing/1/87, and B/Panama/45/90 (n=927) or intramuscular placebo containing physiological saline solution (n=911).

The Efficacy of Influenza Vaccination in Elderly Individuals: A Randomized, Double Blind, Placebo Controlled Trial.

(continued)

Results
:   The incidence of serological influenza was 4% in the vaccine group and 9% in the placebo group (relative risk [RR] 0.5; 95% confidence interval [CI] 0.35–0.61). The incidences of clinical influenza were 2% and 3%, respectively (RR 0.53; 95% CI 0.39–0.73). The effect was strongest for the combination of serological and clinical influenza (RR 0.42; 95% CI 0.23–0.74). The effect was less pronounced for self-reported influenza.

Conclusion
:   In the elderly, influenza vaccination may halve the incidence of serological and clinical influenza (in periods of antigenic drift).

Influenza Vaccination of Health Care Workers in Long-Term-Care Hospitals Reduces the Mortality of Elderly Patients [See Comments]

Title	Influenza vaccination of health care workers in long-term-care hospitals reduces the mortality of elderly patients [see comments].
Authors	Potter J, Stott DJ, Roberts MA, et al.
Reference	J Infect Dis 1997;175(1):1-6.
Disease/ Pathogen	Influenza.
Purpose	To determine if vaccination of health care workers (HCWs), as a strategy for preventing influenza in elderly patients in long-term care, is effective.
Design	Controlled trial.
Patients	During the winter of 1994–1995, 1059 patients in 12 geriatric medical long-term-care sites, randomized for vaccination of HCWs, were studied.
Treatment/ prophylaxis regimen	Vaccination or no vaccination of health care workers.
Results	In hospitals where HCWs were offered vaccination, 653 (61%) of 1078 were vaccinated. Vaccination of HCWs was associated with reductions in total patient mortality, from 17% to 10% (odds ratio [OR] 0.56; 95% confidence interval [CI] 0.4–0.8) and in influenza-like illness (OR 0.57; 95% CI 0.34–0.94). Vaccination of patients was not associated with significant effects on mortality (OR 1.15; 95% CI 0.81–1.64).

Influenza Vaccination of Health Care Workers in Long-Term-Care Hospitals Reduces the Mortality of Elderly Patients [See Comments]

(continued)

Conclusion   Results of this study support recommendations for vaccination against influenza of HCWs in long-term geriatric care. Vaccination of frail elderly long-term-care patients may not give clinically worthwhile benefits.

Effectiveness of Influenza Vaccine in Health Care Professionals: A Randomized Trial.

Title	Effectiveness of influenza vaccine in health care professionals: A randomized trial.
Authors	Wilde JA, McMillan JA, Serwint J, et al.
Reference	JAMA 1999;281:908-913.
Disease/ Pathogen	Influenza.
Purpose	To determine the effectiveness of trivalent influenza vaccine in reducing infection, illness, and absence from work in young, healthy health care professionals.
Design	Randomized, prospective, double blind, controlled trial over 3 consecutive years, from 1992-1993 to 1994-1995.
Patients	264 hospital-based health care professionals without chronic medical problems were recruited; 49 participated for 2 seasons; 24 participated for 3 seasons. The mean age was 28.4 years, 75% were resident physicians, and 57% were women.
Follow-up	Serologically defined influenza infection (four-fold increase in hemagglutination-inhibiting antibodies), days of febrile respiratory illness, and days absent from work.

Effectiveness of Influenza Vaccine in Health Care Professionals: A Randomized Trial.

(continued)

Treatment/ prophylaxis regimen	Participants were randomly assigned to receive either an influenza vaccine or a control (meningococcal vaccine, pneumococcal vaccine, or placebo). Serum samples for antibody assays were collected at the time of vaccination, 1 month after vaccination, and at the end of the influenza season. Active weekly surveillance for illness was conducted during each influenza epidemic period.
Results	The authors conducted 359 person-winters of serologic surveillance (99.4% follow-up) and 4746 person-weeks of illness surveillance (100% follow-up). 24 (13.4%) of 179 control subjects and three (1.7%) of 180 influenza vaccine recipients had serologic evidence of influenza type A or B infection during the study period. Vaccine efficacy against serologically defined infection was 88% for influenza A (95% confidence interval [CI] 47%-97%; p=0.001) and 89% for influenza B (95% CI 14%-99%; p=0.03). Among influenza vaccinees, cumulative days of reported febrile respiratory illness were 28.7 per 100 subjects, compared with 40.6 per 100 subjects in controls (p=0.57) and days of absence were 9.9 per 100 subjects vs 21.1 per 100 subjects in controls (p=0.41).
Conclusion	Influenza vaccine is effective in preventing infection by influenza A and B in health care professionals and may reduce reported days of work absence and febrile respiratory illness. These data support a policy of annual influenza vaccination of health care professionals.

2. Pathogens
bb. Leishmaniasis

Randomised Vaccine Trial of Single Dose of Killed Leishmania Major Plus BCG Against Anthroponotic Cutaneous Leishmaniasis in Bam, Iran

Title	Randomised vaccine trial of single dose of killed Leishmania major plus BCG against anthroponotic cutaneous leishmaniasis in Bam, Iran.
Authors	Sharifi I, FeKri AR, Aflatonian MR, et al.
Reference	Lancet 1998;351:1540–1543.
Disease/ Pathogen	Cutaneous leishmaniasis.
Purpose	To compare a vaccine consisting of a single dose of whole-cell autoclave-killed Leishmania major (ALM) mixed with BCG with BCG alone against anthroponotic (human to human transmission) cutaneous leishmaniasis.
Design	Randomised, double blind trial.
Patients	3637 schoolchildren, aged 6–15 years, with no history of cutaneous leishmaniasis, and no response to a leishmanin skin test.
Follow-up	Safety of the vaccine and the incidence of confirmed cases of cutaneous leishmaniasis were followed up for 2 years.
Treatment/ prophylaxis regimen	Patients were randomly assigned to receive 1 mg ALM mixed with BCG (n=1839), or BCG alone (n=1798).

Randomised Vaccine Trial of Single Dose of Killed Leishmania Major Plus BCG Against Anthroponotic Cutaneous Leishmaniasis in Bam, Iran

(continued)

Results
: Side-effects were those usually associated with BCG vaccination, but tended to persist longer in the ALM + BCG group. After exclusion of four cases occurring within 80 days of vaccination (one in the ALM + BCG group and three in the BCG group), the 2-year incidence of cutaneous leishmaniasis did not differ significantly between vaccine and BCG groups: 2.8% vs 3.3%, respectively (total cases 112). A sex-stratified analysis showed that in boys the vaccine conferred a protective efficacy of 18% and 78% for the first and second years, respectively—a crude 2-year overall protection of 55% (95% confidence interval [CI] 19%–75%, p<0.01). In the first 9 months after vaccination, there was a non-significant excess of cases in the ALM + BCG group (25 vs 16), whereas the incidence of cutaneous leishmaniasis thereafter was significantly reduced in the ALM + BCG group (27 vs 44, p<0.05).

Conclusion
: A single dose of ALM + BCG was safe and more immunogenic than BCG alone, as measured by leishmanin skin test. The exact reason for the apparent protective effect of the vaccine in boys is unknown, and may be a chance finding. However, since boys are more exposed to the infection, which is indicated by higher disease prevalence in boys in this study population, the preferential protective effect in boys may have resulted from a greater booster effect produced by repeated exposure to infected sandflies. Booster injections or alternative adjuvants should be tried to improve the potential efficacy of this vaccine.

Short-Course, Low-Dose Amphotericin B Lipid Complex Therapy for Visceral Leishmaniasis Unresponsive to Antimony

Title	Short-course, low-dose amphotericin B lipid complex therapy for visceral leishmaniasis unresponsive to antimony.
Authors	Sundar S, Agrawal NK, Sinha PR, et al.
Reference	Ann Intern Med 1997;127:133–137.
Disease/ Pathogen	Visceral Leishmaiasis.
Purpose	To determine the efficacy and minimal effective dose of short-course therapy with amphotericin B lipid complex in visceral leishmaniasis.
Design	Randomized, open label study.
Patients	60 patients with active infection, who had not responded to or who had relapse after receiving conventional (>30 days) treatment with pentavalent antimony.
Follow-up	Mean of 11.2± 0.2 months (range, 10–13 months).
Treatment/ prophylaxis regimen	Intravenous amphotericin B lipid complex was given once daily for 5 consecutive days by 2-hour infusion. Patients were randomly assigned to receive 1, 2, or 3 mg/kg of body weight per day (total doses of 5, 10, or 15 mg/kg, respectively).

Results	All 60 patients responded to 5 days of treatment. 14 days after therapy, all patients had parasite-free splenic aspirates and were considered to have an apparent clinical and parasitologic response. 6 months after therapy, definitive responses were documented in 16 of 19 (84% [95% confidence interval [CI] 60%-97%]), 18 of 20 (90% [CI 68%-99%]), and 21 of 21 (100% [CI 84%-100%]) patients who received total doses of 5, 10, and 15 mg/kg, respectively.
Conclusion	Short-course therapy with low-dose amphotericin B lipid complex is effective for visceral leishmaniasis and is an important therapeutic alternative in the management of this serious intracellular protozoal infection.

Safety and Efficacy of Intravenous Sodium Stibogluconate in the Treatment of Leishmaniasis: Recent U.S. Military Experience.

Title	Safety and efficacy of intravenous sodium stibogluconate in the treatment of leishmaniasis: Recent U.S. military experience.
Authors	Aronson NE, Wortmann GW, Johnson SC, et al.
Reference	Clin Infect Dis 1998;27(6):1457–1464.
Disease/ Pathogen	Leishmaniasis.
Purpose	To determine the safety and efficacy of intravenous sodium stibogluconate (SSG) in the treatment of leishmaniasis.
Design	Prospective trial.
Patients	96 U.S. Department of Defense health care beneficiaries with parasitologically confirmed leishmaniasis.
Follow-up	Prospective follow-up for 1 year.
Treatment/ prophylaxis regimen	Patients received sodium stibogluconate at a dosage of 20 mg/(kg.d) for either 20 days (for cutaneous disease) or 28 days (for visceral, mucosal, or viscerotropic disease).

Safety and Efficacy of Intravenous Sodium Stibogluconate
in the Treatment of Leishmaniasis:
Recent U.S. Military Experience.

(continued)

Results

One patient was infected with human immunodeficiency virus; otherwise, comorbidity was absent. Clinical cure occurred in 91% of 83 cases of cutaneous disease and 93% of 13 cases of visceral/viscerotropic disease. Adverse effects were common and necessitated interruption of treatment in 28% of cases, but they were generally reversible. These included arthralgias and myalgias (58%), pancreatitis (97%), transaminitis (67%), headache (22%), hematologic suppression (44%), and rash (9%). No subsequent mucosal leishmaniasis was identified, and there were no deaths attributable to SSG or leishmaniasis.

Conclusion

Sodium stibogluconate appears to be effective in the treatment of cutaneous and visceral leishmaniasis; however, side effects such as pancreatitis and arthralgias are common.

Short-Course Treatment of Visceral Leishmaniasis with Liposomal Amphotericin B (AmBisome)

Title	Short-course treatment of visceral leishmaniasis with liposomal amphotericin B (AmBisome).
Authors	Davidson RN, di Martino L, Gradoni L, et al.
Reference	Clin Infect Dis 1996;22(6):938–943.
Disease/ Pathogen	Visceral leishmaniasis caused by Leishmania infantum.
Purpose	To determine the efficacy of liposomal amphoteracin B (AmBisome) for the treatment of visceral leishmaniasis (VL) in immunocompetent patients.
Design	Prospective study.
Patients	88 immunocompetent patients (56 children) with VL caused by L. infantum.
Treatment/ prophylaxis regimen	Patients received liposomal amphotericin B of varying dosages.
Results	13 patients received 4 mg/kg on days 1–5 and 10 (total dose, 24 mg/kg), and all were cured; 42 received 3 mg/kg on days 1–5 and 10 (18 mg/kg), and 41 were cured; 32 received 3 mg/kg on days 1–4 and 10 (15 mg/kg), and 29 were cured (amastigotes were not cleared from one child, and two relapsed). One adult was cured with a total dose of 12mg/kg. The four children who were not cured received 3 mg/kg for 10 days; none had further relapses. There were no significant adverse events.

Conclusion   For VL due to L. infantum, a total dose of AmBisome of ≥20 mg/kg, given in ≥5 doses of 3-4 mg/kg over ≥10 days can be effective.

Effect of Treatment with Interferon-Gamma Alone in Visceral Leishmaniasis

Title	Effect of treatment with interferon-gamma alone in visceral leishmaniasis.
Authors	Sundar S, Murray HW.
Reference	J Infect Dis. 172(6):1627–1629, 1995 Dec.
Disease/ Pathogen	Visceral leishmaniasis.
Purpose	To determine the effect of cytokine immunotherapy alone for the treatment of visceral leishmaniasis.
Design	Prospective study.
Patients	9 patients with kala-azar.
Treatment/ prophylaxis regimen	Patients were treated with IFN-gamma before receiving antimony.
Results	After 20 days of IFN-gamma therapy, four patients showed no parasitologic response; in the remaining five patients. However, splenic aspirate parasite scores declined from 4.2±0.2 to 1.2±0.5 (mean +/- SE).
Conclusion	These results indicate that treatment with IFN-gamma alone can induce visceral antileishmanial activity. However, the limited efficacy in this uncontrolled pilot trial suggests that the therapeutic role of IFN-gamma in kala-azar is that of an adjunct to conventional antimony treatment.

2. Pathogens

cc. Leprosy

Powerful Bactericidal Activities of Clarithromycin and Minocycline Against Mycobacterium Leprae in Lepromatous Leprosy

Title	Powerful bactericidal activities of clarithromycin and minocycline against Mycobacterium leprae in lepromatous leprosy.
Authors	Ji B, Jamet P, Perani EG, et al.
Reference	J Infect Dis 1993;168(1):188–190.
Disease/ Pathogen	Lepromatous leprosy.
Purpose	To determine the bactericidal activities of clarithromycin and minocycline against M. leprae in lepromatous leprosy.
Design	Randomized trial.
Patients	36 patients with newly diagnosed lepromatous leprosy.
Follow-up	56 days.
Treatment/ prophylaxis regimen	Patients were randomly assigned to three groups with minocycline (100 mg daily), clarithromycin (500 mg daily), or clarithromycin (500 mg) plus minocycline (100 mg daily).

Powerful Bactericidal Activities of Clarithromycin and Minocycline Against Mycobacterium Leprae in Lepromatous Leprosy

(continued)

Results
All groups had rapid and remarkable clinical improvement and significant decline of the bacterial and morphologic indices in skin smears during treatment. More than 99% and >99.9% of the viable M. leprae had been killed by 28 and 56 days of treatment, respectively, as measured by inoculation of organisms recovered from skin samples, taken before and during treatment, into the footpads of immunocompetent and nude mice. Clinical improvement and bactericidal activity did not differ significantly among the three groups. Adverse reactions were rare and mild, and no laboratory abnormality was detected during the trial.

Conclusion
Both clarithromycin and minocycline displayed powerful bactericidal activities against M. leprae in leprosy patients and may be considered important components of new multidrug regimens for the treatment of multibacillary leprosy.

2. Pathogens

dd. Lyme Disease

A Vaccine Consisting of Recombinant Borrelia Burgdorferi Outer-Surface Protein A to Prevent Lyme Disease

Title	A vaccine consisting of recombinant borrelia burgdorferi outer-surface protein A to prevent Lyme disease.
Authors	Sigal LH, Zahradnik JM, Lavin P, et al.
Reference	N Engl J Med 1998;339:216–222.
Disease/ Pathogen	Lyme disease.
Purpose	To evaluate the protective efficacy of a 30 mg dose of vaccine in adults at risk for B. burgdorferi infection.
Design	Randomized, double blind, placebo controlled, multicenter.
Patients	A total of 10,305 subjects (age range, 18–92 years of age) were enrolled at 14 study sites in areas of the United States in which Lyme disease was endemic and were randomly assigned to receive two doses of either 30 mg of outer-surface protein A (OspA) vaccine or placebo, given one month apart, according to a preset randomization schedule.
Follow-up	The subjects were observed during the two seasons in which the risk of disease transmission was greatest, irrespective of whether they had received the booster dose.
Treatment/ prophylaxis regimen	Two doses of either 30 mg of OspA vaccine or placebo, given one month apart, according to a preset randomization schedule.

Results

The efficacy of the vaccine was 68% in the first year of the study in the entire population, and 92% in the second year, among the 3745 subjects who received the third injection. The vaccine was well tolerated. There was a higher incidence of mild, self-limited local and systemic reactions in the vaccine group, but only during the 7 days after vaccination. There was no significant increase in the frequency of arthritis or neurologic events in vaccine recipients.

Conclusion

In this study, OspA vaccine was safe and effective in the prevention of Lyme disease.

Vaccination Against Lyme Disease with Recombinant Borrelia Burgdorferi Outer-Surface Lipoprotein A with Adjuvant

Title	Vaccination against Lyme disease with recombinant Borrelia burgdorferi outer-surface lipoprotein A with adjuvant.
Authors	Steere AC, Sikand VK, Meurice F, et al.
Reference	N Engl J Med 1998;339:209–215.
Disease/ Pathogen	Lyme disease.
Purpose	To determine the efficacy, safety, and immunogenicity of an outer-surface lipoprotein A (OspA) with adjuvant vaccine.
Design	Randomized, double blind, placebo controlled, multicenter.
Patients	10,936 subjects (age, 15–70 years) were enrolled in the study in 10 states where Lyme disease is endemic.
Follow-up	20 months after study entry.
Treatment/ prophylaxis regimen	Injection of either recombinant B. burgdorferi OspA with adjuvant or placebo at enrollment and 1 and 12 months later.

Vaccination Against Lyme Disease with Recombinant Borrelia Burgdorferi Outer-Surface Lipoprotein A with Adjuvant

(continued)

Results   In the first year, after two injections, 22 subjects in the vaccine group, and 43 in the placebo group, contracted definite Lyme disease (p=0.009); vaccine efficacy was 49% (95% confidence interval [CI] 15%-69%). In the second year, after the third injection, 16 vaccine recipients and 66 placebo recipients, contracted definite Lyme disease (p<0.001); vaccine efficacy was 76% (95% CI 58%-86%). The efficacy of the vaccine in preventing asymptomatic infection was 83% in the first year, and 100% in the second year. Injection of the vaccine was associated with mild-to-moderate local or systemic reactions lasting a median of 3 days.

Conclusion   Three injections of vaccine prevented most definite cases of Lyme disease or asymptomatic B. burgdorferi infection.

Bloodstream Invasion in Early Lyme Disease: Results From a Prospective, Controlled, Blinded Study Using the Polymerase Chain Reaction.

Title	Bloodstream invasion in early Lyme disease: Results from a prospective, controlled, blinded study using the polymerase chain reaction.
Authors	Goodman JL, Bradley JF, Ross AE et al.
Reference	Am J Med 1995;99(1):6–12.
Disease/ Pathogen	Lyme disease.
Purpose	The purposes of this study were to determine (1) the optimal techniques for and potential diagnostic usefulness of the polymerase chain reaction (PCR) in early Lyme disease; and (2) the true frequency and clinical correlates of PCR-documented blood-borne infection in the dissemination of Lyme disease.
Design	Prospective, controlled, blinded study of PCR, culture, and serology on fractionated blood samples.
Patients	105 patients; 76 with physician-diagnosed erythema migrans and 29 controls.
Follow-up	Clinical characteristics of the patients were obtained with a standardized data entry form and correlated with results of the laboratory studies.

(continued)

Results	Only 4 of the 76 (5.3%) patients with erythema migrans were culture positive. However, 14 of 76 (18.4%) had spirochetemia documented by PCR of their plasma. None of 29 contols were PCR or culture positive (p=0.007, vs patients), PCR-documented spirochetemia correlated with clinical evidence of disseminated disease; 10 of 33 patients (30.3%) with systemic symptom(s) were PCR-positive compared to 4 of 43 (9.3%) without such evidence (p=0.02). PCR positivity was more frequent among patients with each of four specific symptoms: Fever, arthralgia, myalgia, and headache (all p<0.05). A higher total number of symptoms (median 2.5 in PCR-positive patients vs 0 in PCR-negative controls; p<0.01) and the presence of multiple skin lesions (37.5% of patients with multiple, vs 13.3% of patients with single lesions [p=0.04] were also correlated with PCR positivity. Patients with both systemic symptoms and multiple skin lesions had a 40% PCR-positivity rate. However, four of 42 (9.5%) asymptomatic patients with only single erythema migrans lesions were also PCR positive. In multivariate analysis using logistic regression, the number of systemic symptoms was the strongest independent predictor of PCR positivity (p=0.004).
Conclusion	PCR detection of B. burgdorfei is ar least three times more sensitive than culture for identifying spirochetemia in early Lyme disease, and may be useful in rapid diagnosis. PCR positivity significantly correlates with clinical evidence of disease dissemination. Bloodstream invasion is an important and common mechanism for the dissemination of the Lyme disease spirochete.

2. Pathogens

ee. Malaria

Effect of Paracetamol on Parasite Clearance Time in Plasmodium Falciparum Malaria

Title	Effect of paracetamol on parasite clearance time in Plasmodium falciparum malaria.
Authors	Brandts CH, Ndjave M, Graninger W, et al.
Reference	Lancet 1997;350:704–709.
Disease/ Pathogen	Plasmodium falciparum.
Purpose	To determine the effectiveness of paracetamol to reduce fever.
Design	Randomized, controlled trial.
Patients	50 children with P. falciparum malaria.
Follow-up	Rectal body temperature and parasitaemia were recorded every 6 h for 4 days. Plasma concentrations and inducible concentrations of tumor necrosis factor (TNF) and interleukin-6 were measured every 24 h. In addition, production of oxygen radicals was measured in both groups.
Treatment/ prophylaxis regimen	Pateints were treated with intravenous quinine, and received either mechanical antipyresis alone, or in combination with paracetamol.

Effect of Paracetamol on Parasite Clearance Time in Plasmodium Falciparum Malaria

(continued)

Results   The mean fever clearance time was 32 h for children treated with paracetamol, and 43 h for those who received
mechanical antipyresis alone. However, this 11 h difference was not significant (95% confidence interval [CI]
-2-24 h; p=0.176). Parasite clearance time was significantly prolonged in patients who received paracetamol
with a difference of 16 h (8-24 h; p=0.004). Plasma concentrations of TNF and interleukin-6 were similar in both
groups during the study. However, the induced concentrations of TNF, and the production of oxygen radicals,
were significantly lower in children treated with paracetamol than those who received mechanical antipyresis
alone.

Conclusion   These data suggest that paracetamol has no antipyretic
benefits over mechanical antipyresis alone in P. falciparum
malaria. Moreover, paracetamol prolongs parasite clearance time, possibly by decreased production of TNF and
oxygen radicals.

2. Pathogens
ff. Measles

Measles Re-Immunization in Children Seronegative After Initial Immunization

Title	Measles re-immunization in children seronegative after initial immunization.
Authors	Poland GA, Jacobson RM, Thampy AM, et al.
Reference	JAMA 1997;277(14):1156–1158.
Disease/ Pathogen	Measles.
Purpose	To evaluate the success of measles re-immunization in children without measles antibody after the initial dose of measles vaccine.
Design	Prospective, clinical trial.
Patients	A total of 130 healthy, white, Innu, and Inuit schoolchildren. All subjects had received the post-1980 Moraten measles vaccine 4–11 years earlier.
Follow-up	Measles antibody was measured a minimum of 6 weeks later using a whole-virus IgG measles-specific enzyme-linked immunoassay (EIA).
Treatment/ prophylaxis regimen	Children previously identified as measles antibody seronegative or equivocal after 1 dose of measles vaccine were entered into the trial and re-immunized.

Results

Of the 130 children re-immunized, 106 (81.5%) became measles antibody seropositive, but 24 children (18.5%) remained seronegative. Younger age at initial immunization (<13 months vs ≥13 months) was significantly associated with lack of seropositive antibody levels following reimmunization (odds ratio 3.9; 95% confidence interval 1.5–9.7). In addition, antibody levels after re-immunization were significantly reduced with increasing time since initial immunization (p=0.001).

Conclusion

After two doses of measles vaccine, 98.2% of all subjects in this study were seropositive for measles antibody, despite the fact that almost 20% of children did not have measurable antibodies 4–11 years following a first dose. These findings suggest that the current public health policy recommending a 2-dose measles immunization strategy, with the second dose given at school entry, will provide high levels of immunity in the community.

2. Pathogens
gg. Pertussis

A Controlled Trial of Two Acellular Vaccines and One Whole-Cell Vaccine against Pertussis

Title	A controlled trial of two acellular vaccines and one whole-cell vaccine against pertussis.
Authors	Greco D, Salmaso S, Mastrantonio P, et al.
Reference	N Engl J Med 1996;334:341–348.
Disease/ Pathogen	Pertussis.
Purpose	To examine the efficacy of each vaccine, given at 2, 4, and 6 months of age, in preventing laboratory-confirmed clinical pertussis.
Design	Prospective, randomized, clinical trial, multicenter.
Patients	14,751 children.
Follow-up	17 months
Treatment/ prophylaxis regimen	Vaccination at 2, 4, and 6 months of age with an acellular pertussis vaccine together with diphtheria and tetanus toxoids (DTP); a DTP vaccine containing whole-cell pertussis (manufactured by Connaught Laboratories); or diphtheria and tetanus toxoids without pertussis (DT).

A Controlled Trial of Two Acellular Vaccines and One Whole-Cell Vaccine against Pertussis

(continued)

Results   For both of the acellular DTP vaccines, the efficacy was 84% (95% confidence intervals [CI] 76%-89% for SmithKline DTP and 76%-90% for Biocine DTP), whereas the efficacy of the whole-cell DTP vaccine was only 36% (95% CI 14%-52%). The antibody responses were greater to the acellular vaccines than to the whole-cell vaccine. Local and systemic adverse events were significantly more frequent after the administration of the whole-cell vaccine. For the acellular vaccines, the frequency of adverse events was similar to that in the control (DT) group.

Conclusion   The two acellular DTP vaccines we studied were safe, immunogenic, and efficacious against pertussis, whereas the efficacy of the whole-cell DTP vaccine was unexpectedly low.

2. Pathogens

hh. Pseudomonas Infections

Title	Prevention of chronic Pseudomonas aeruginosa colonisation in cystic fibrosis by early treatment.
Authors	Valerius NH, Koch C, Hoiby N.
Reference	Lancet 1991;338:725–726.
Disease/ Pathogen	Pseudomonas aeruginosa.
Purpose	To assess whether chronic pulmonary colonisation with P. aeruginosa in cystic fibrosis is preventable.
Design	Randomized trial.
Patients	26 patients who had never received anti-pseudomonas chemotherapy.
Follow-up	27 months.
Treatment/ prophylaxis regimen	Patients received either no anti-pseudomonas chemotherapy or oral ciprofloxacin and aerosol inhalations of colistin twice daily for 3 weeks, whenever P. aeruginosa was isolated from routine sputum cultures.
Results	During the trial, infection with P. aeruginosa became chronic in significantly fewer treated than untreated subjects (2 [14%] vs 7 [58%]; p<0.05) and there were significantly fewer P. aeruginosa isolates in routine sputum cultures in the treated group (49/214 [23%] vs 64/158 [41%]; p=0.0006).

Conclusion   Chronic colonisation with P. aeruginosa can be prevented
                in cystic fibrosis by early institution of anti-pseudomonas
                chemotherapy.

Title	Ceftazidime monotherapy vs ceftriaxone/tobramycin for serious hospital-acquired, gram-negative infections.
Authors	Rubinstein E, Lode H, Grassi C.
Reference	Clin Infect Dis 1995;20(5):1217–1228.
Disease/ Pathogen	Hospital-acquired, gram-negative infections.
Purpose	To compare ceftazidime monotherapy with ceftriaxone/tobramycin in patients with serious hospital-acquired infections.
Design	Prospective, randomized, clinical trial.
Patients	580 patients with serious hospital-acquired infections.
Treatment/ prophylaxis regimen	Patients received either ceftazidime monotherapy or ceftriaxone/tobramycin.

(continued)

Results

One half of the patients had an underlying disease with a rapidly or ultimately fatal prognosis; 40% were nursed in intensive care units. Clinical response among patients with pneumonia (73% in the ceftazidime group vs 65% in the ceftriaxone/tobramycin group), septicemia (73% vs 59%), and complicated urinary tract infections (80% vs 76%) showed that there were no significant differences in efficacy between the two regimens. Pseudomonas aeruginosa was the most prevalent pathogen, and was effectively eradicated by both treatments. The odds of bacteriologic cure with either study regimen were equal. Mortality was similar in both treatment groups. Ceftazidime monotherapy was not associated with a higher incidence of development of resistance or superinfection. Both regimens were well tolerated; no patients receiving ceftazidime evidenced nephrotoxicity, compared with nine who received the combination.

Conclusion

The authors conclude that ceftazidime may be used as monotherapy in the empirical treatment of patients with serious nosocomial infections.

2. Pathogens

ii. Respiratory Syncytial Virus Infection

A Controlled Trial of Aerosolized Ribavirin in Infants Receiving Mechanical Ventilation for Severe Respiratory Syncytial Virus Infection

Title	A controlled trial of aerosolized ribavirin in infants receiving mechanical ventilation for severe respiratory syncytial virus infection.
Authors	Smith DW, Frankel LR, Mathers LH, et al.
Reference	New Engl J Med 1991;325:24–29.
Disease/ Pathogen	Respiratory syncyctial virus infection.
Purpose	To determine if ribavirin can benefit infants with severe respiratory syncytial virus disease who require mechanical ventilation.
Design	Randomized, double blind, placebo controlled.
Treatment/ prophylaxis regimen	Ribavirin (20 mg per milliliter) administered continuously in aerosolized form to infants receiving mechanical ventilation for respiratory failure that was caused by documented respiratory syncytial virus infection.

A Controlled Trial of Aerosolized Ribavirin in Infants Receiving Mechanical Ventilation for Severe Respiratory Syncytial Virus Infection

(continued)

Results

Of the 28 infants (mean [±SD] age, 1.4±1.7 months) enrolled, seven had underlying diseases predisposing them to severe infection (mean age, 3±2.6 months), and 21 were previously normal (mean age, 0.8±0.9 month). Among the 14 infants who received ribavirin, the mean duration of mechanical ventilation was 4.9 days (as compared with 9.9 days among the 14 who received placebo; p=0.01), and the mean length of supplemental oxygen use was 8.7 days (as compared with 13.5 days; p=0.01). The mean length of the hospital stay was 13.3 days after treatment with ribavirin and 15.0 with placebo (p=0.04). When only the 21 previously normal infants were considered, the mean length of the hospital stay was 9 days for the ribavirin recipients, and 15.3 days for those who received placebo (p=0.005).

Conclusion

In infants who require mechanical ventilation because of severe respiratory syncytial virus infection, treatment with aerosolized ribavirin decreases the duration of mechanical ventilation, oxygen treatment, and the hospital stay.

2. Pathogens

jj. Rotavirus Infections

Efficacy of the Rhesus Rotavirus-Based Quadrivalent Vaccine in Infants and Young Children in Venezuela

Title	Efficacy of the rhesus rotavirus-based quadrivalent vaccine in infants and young children in Venezuela.
Authors	Perez-Schael I, Guntinas MJ, Perez M, et al.
Reference	N Engl J Med 1997;337:1181–1187.
Disease/ Pathogen	Rotavirus infection.
Purpose	To evaluate the efficacy of the vaccine against dehydration as the primary end point.
Design	Randomized, double blind, placebo controlled, multicenter.
Patients	2207 infants.
Follow-up	19–20 months of passive surveillance
Treatment/ prophylaxis regimen	Three oral doses of the quadrivalent rotavirus vaccine (4 x 10[5]) plaque-forming units per dose) or placebo at about 2, 3, and 4 months of age.

Results

The vaccine was safe, although 15% of the vaccinated infants had febrile episodes (rectal temperature, greater/equal 38.1 degrees C) during the 6 days after the first dose, as compared with 7% of the controls (p<0.001). However, the vaccine gave 88% protection against severe diarrhea caused by rotavirus and 75% protection against dehydration, and produced a 70% reduction in hospital admissions. Overall, the efficacy of the vaccine against a first episode of rotavirus diarrhea was 48%. Horizontal transmission of vaccine virus was demonstrated in 15% of the vaccine recipients and 13% of the placebo recipients with rotavirus-positive diarrhea.

Conclusion

In this study in a developing country, the quadrivalent rhesus rotavirus-based vaccine induced a high level of protection against severe diarrheal illness caused by rotavirus.

Title	Evaluation of rhesus rotavirus monovalent and tetravalent re-assortant vaccines in U.S. children.
Authors	Bernstein DI, Glass RI, Rodgers G, et al.
Reference	JAMA 1995;273:1191–1196.
Disease/ Pathogen	Rotavirus.
Purpose	To determine the safety and relative efficacy of two re-assortant rhesus rotavirus vaccines over two rotavirus seasons.
Design	A prospective, double masked, placebo controlled trial.
Patients	A total of 1006 healthy infants between 4 and 26 weeks of age were enrolled, and 898 received three doses of vaccine or placebo.
Follow-up	Reactogenicity was determined by comparing the incidence of fever, diarrhea, and/or vomiting for 5 days after each dose of vaccine. Rotavirus IgA and neutralizing antibody to rhesus rotavirus and four rotavirus serotypes were measured in a subset of subjects. Relative efficacy was determined by comparing the incidence of rotavirus gastroenteritis after three doses of vaccine or placebo over two rotavirus seasons.
Treatment/ prophylaxis regimen	Three doses of vaccine or placebo.

Results
Adverse reactions were mild and limited to a small but significant increase in the incidence of fever after the first dose of tetravalent but not monovalent vaccine. The relative efficacy against rotavirus disease over the 2 years of observation was 40% (98.3% confidence interval [CI] 7% to 62%) for the monovalent and 57% (98.3% CI 29%-74%) for the tetravalent vaccine. In post hoc analyses, the relative efficacy against very severe rotavirus gastroenteritis was 73%, and 82% for monovalent and tetravalent vaccine recipients, respectively. Also, a 67% and 78% reduction in medical visits for rotavirus gastroenteritis was observed. Both vaccines protected against disease caused by serotype 1 rotavirus, but only the tetravalent vaccine reduced the incidence of disease caused by non-serotype 1 rotavirus infection detected in the second season. It is unclear, however, whether this result represents serotype-specific protection or a difference in the duration of protection.

Conclusion
Vaccination with both vaccines was safe and significantly reduced the incidence of rotavirus gastroenteritis, but only the tetravalent vaccine provided protection against disease caused by non-serotype 1 rotaviruses during the second year of follow-up.

Randomised, Placebo Controlled Trial of Rhesus-Human Re-Assortant Rotavirus Vaccine for Prevention of Severe Rotavirus Gastroenteritis

Title	Randomised, placebo controlled trial of rhesus-human re-assortant rotavirus vaccine for prevention of severe rotavirus gastroenteritis.
Authors	Joensuu J, Koskenniemi E, Pang XL, et al.
Reference	Lancet 1997;350:1205–1209.
Disease/ Pathogen	Rotavirus.
Purpose	To assess the efficacy of rhesus-human re-assortant rotavirus tetravalent vaccine (RRV-TV) against severe rotavirus gastroenteritis
Design	Randomized, double blind, placebo controlled trial.
Patients	2398 children were enrolled and received at least one dose of RRV-TV (n=1191) or placebo (n=1207). The primary efficacy analysis was based on children who received three doses of RRV-TV (n=1128) or placebo (n=1145).
Follow-up	The children were followed up for one or two rotavirus epidemic seasons. The main outcome measure was protection against severe rotavirus gastroenteritis (score ≥11 on a 20-point severity scale).
Treatment/ prophylaxis regimen	Placebo or RRV-TV (titer $4 \times 10(5)$ plaque-forming units) was given to infants at ages 2, 3, and 5 months.

Randomised, Placebo Controlled Trial of Rhesus-Human Re-Assortant Rotavirus Vaccine for Prevention of Severe Rotavirus Gastroenteritis

(continued)

Results
256 episodes of rotavirus gastroenteritis occurred at any time during the study; 65 were among 1191 RRV-TV recipients, and 191 among 1207 placebo recipients (vaccine efficacy 66% [95% confidence interval [CI] 55–74]; intention-to-treat analysis). 226 episodes were included in the primary efficacy analysis of fully vaccinated children (54 among 1128 RRV-TV recipients, 172 among 1145 placebo recipients; vaccine efficacy 68% [57–76]). 100 episodes were severe, eight in RRV-TV recipients and 92 in placebo recipients (vaccine efficacy 91% [82–96]).

Conclusion
RRV-TV vaccine was highly effective against severe rotavirus gastroenteritis in young children. Incorporation of this vaccine into routine immunisation schedules of infants could reduce severe rotavirus gastroenteritis by 90%, and severe gastroenteritis of all causes in young children by 60%.

2. Pathogens
kk. Salmonellosis

Ciprofloxacin and Trimethoprim-Sulfamethoxazole Vs Placebo in Acute Uncomplicated Salmonella enteritis: A Double Blind Trial.

Title	Ciprofloxacin and trimethoprim-sulfamethoxazole vs placebo in acute uncomplicated Salmonella enteritis: A double blind trial.
Authors	Sanchez C, Garcia-Restoy E, Garau J, et al.
Reference	J Infect Dis 1993;168(5):1304–1307.
Disease/ Pathogen	Salmonella.
Purpose	The role of ciprofloxacin and trimethoprim-sulfamethoxazole (TMP-SMZ) was evaluated in empiric treatment of uncomplicated Salmonella enteritis.
Design	Comparative, double blind trial.
Patients	There were 65 evaluable patients with acute, uncomplicated, culture-confirmed Salmonella enteritis.
Treatment/ prophylaxis regimen	Patients were randomized to receive ciprofloxacin (500 mg), TMP-SMZ (160/800 mg), or placebo orally twice daily for 5 days.

Ciprofloxacin and Trimethoprim-Sulfamethoxazole Vs Placebo in Acute Uncomplicated Salmonella enteritis: A Double Blind Trial.

(continued)

Results

Duration of diarrhea, abdominal pain, or vomiting and time to defervescence were not significantly different for patients treated with ciprofloxacin, TMP-SMZ, or placebo. There also were no significant differences with respect to full resolution of symptoms for ciprofloxacin vs placebo (point estimate, 0.2 days; 95% confidence interval [CI] -0.5-0.9 days) or for TMP-SMZ vs placebo (point estimate 0.2 days; 95% CI -1-0.6 days). The rate of clearance of salmonellae from stools was not significantly different among the groups.

2. Pathogens

11. Schistosomiasis

Double Blind, Placebo Controlled Study of Concurrent Administration of Albendazole and Praziquantel in Schoolchildren with Schistosomiasis and Geohelminths

Title	Double blind, placebo controlled study of concurrent administration of albendazole and praziquantel in schoolchildren with schistosomiasis and geohelminths.
Authors	Olds GR, King C, Hewlett J, et al.
Reference	J Infect Dis 1999;179(4):996–1003.
Disease/ Pathogen	Schistosomiasis.
Purpose	To determine the efficacy of the concurrent administration of albendazole and praziquantel in children with schistosomiasis and geohelminths.
Design	Double blind, placebo controlled, multicenter study.
Patients	1500 children with high prevalences of geohelminths and schistosomiasis. The study sites were in China and the Philippines, including 2 strains of Schistosoma japonicum, and two different regions of Kenya, one each with endemic Schistosoma mansoni or Schistosoma haematobium.
Treatment/ prophylaxis regimen	Concurrent administration of albendazole and praziquantel or placebo.

***Double Blind, Placebo Controlled Study of Concurrent
Administration of Albendazole and Praziquantel in
Schoolchildren with Schistosomiasis and Geohelminths***

(continued)

Results	Neither medication affected the cure rate of the other. There was no difference between the side effect rate from albendazole or the double placebo. Praziquantel-treated children had more nausea, abdominal pain, and headache, but these side effects were statistically more common in children with schistosomiasis, suggesting a strong influence of dying parasites. The subjects were followed for 6 months for changes in infection status, growth parameters, hemoglobin, and schistosomiasis morbidity.
Conclusion	In all four sites, a significant 6-month increase in serum hemoglobin was observed in children who received praziquantel, strongly supporting population-based mass treatment.

2. Pathogens
mm. Shigellosis

Treatment of Shigellosis: III. Comparison of One- or Two-dose Ciprofloxacin With Standard 5-Day Therapy.
Treatment of Shigellosis: IV. Cefixime Is Ineffective in Shigellosis in Adults.
Treatment of Shigellosis: V. Comparison of Azithromycin and Ciprofloxacin: A Double Blind, Randomized, Controlled Trial.

Title	Treatment of shigellosis: III. Comparison of one- or two-dose ciprofloxacin with standard 5-day therapy. Treatment of Shigellosis: IV. Cefixime is ineffective in shigellosis in adults. Treatment of Shigellosis: V. comparison of azithromycin and ciprofloxacin: A double blind, randomized, controlled trial.
Authors	Bennish ML, Salam MA, Khan WA, et al. Salam MA, Seas C, Khan WA, et al. Khan WA, Seas C, Dhar U, et al.
Reference	Ann Intern Med 1992;117:727–734. Ann Intern Med 1995;123:505–508. Ann Intern Med 1997;126:697–703.
Disease/ Pathogen	Shigellosis.
Purpose	To determine whether a single dose, or two doses, of ciprofloxacin are as effective as 5-day, 10-dose therapy for the treatment of shigellosis in adult men who are moderately to severely ill. To compare the efficacy of cefixime with that of pivamdinocillin in the treatment of adults with acute dysentery caused by shigella infection. To determine the efficacy of azithromycin in the treatment of shigellosis.

Treatment of Shigellosis: III. Comparison of One- or Two-dose Ciprofloxacin With Standard 5-Day Therapy. Treatment of Shigellosis: IV. Cefixime Is Ineffective in Shigellosis in Adults. Treatment of Shigellosis: V. Comparison of Azithromycin and Ciprofloxacin: A Double Blind, Randomized, Controlled Trial.

(continued)

Design	Randomized, double blind clinical trial.
Patients	A total of 128 adult men with dysentery of less than 96 hours duration. All had shigella organisms isolated from a culture of stool. 30 men with dysentery lasting 72 hours or less. 70 men with shigellosis that had lasted 72 hours or less.
Follow-up	6 days. 6 days. 5 days.
Treatment/ prophylaxis regimen	Patients were randomly assigned to receive either a single 1-gram dose of ciprofloxacin at admission to the study (single-dose group; n=40), a 1-gram dose of ciprofloxacin at admission and 24 hours later (2-dose group; n=43), or 500 mg of ciprofloxacin every 12 hours for 5 days (10 dose group; n=35). Patients were randomly assigned to receive either 400 mg of cefixime every 24 hours (n=5) or 400 mg of pivamdinocillin every 6 hours (n=15) for 5 days. Patients stayed in the hospital for 6 days. 34 patients were randomly assigned to receive 500 mg of azithromycin on study day 1, followed by 250 mg once daily for 4 days; 36 patients were assigned to receive 500 mg of ciprofloxacin every 12 hours for 5 days.

Treatment of Shigellosis: III. Comparison of One- or Two-dose Ciprofloxacin With Standard 5-Day Therapy. Treatment of Shigellosis: IV. Cefixime Is Ineffective in Shigellosis in Adults. Treatment of Shigellosis: V. Comparison of Azithromycin and Ciprofloxacin: A Double Blind, Randomized, Controlled Trial.

(continued)

Results

There were no treatment failures in the 78 patients infected with species of shigella other than Shigella dysenteriae type 1. Among the 40 patients infected with S. dysenteriae type 1, treatment failed in four of the 10 patients who received single-dose therapy, two of the 15 patients who received 2-dose therapy, and none of the 15 patients who received 10-dose therapy (p=0.017, single-dose therapy group, compared with 10-dose group; p=0.15 for the single-dose group, compared with the 2-dose group; p>0.2 for the 2-dose group, compared with the 10-dose group).

Therapy failed in seven (47%) patients given cefixime, but in none of the patients given pivamdinocillin (p=0.006). Patients given cefixime had longer duration of fever (median, 6 hours, compared with 0 hours, p=0.019), longer duration of the period with dysenteric stools (median, 4 days compared with 1 day, p=0.001), and more stools during the 6 study days (median 65, compared with 28, p=0.002) than patients treated with pivamdinocillin. Bacteriologic failure of therapy occurred in 60% of patients (nine of 15) given cefixime and 13% of those (two of 15) given pivamdinocillin (p=0.009).

Therapy was clinically successful in 28 (82%) patients who received azithromycin, and 32 (89%) patients who received ciprofloxacin (difference -7% [95% confidence interval (CI) -23%–10%]). Therapy was bacteriologically successful in 32 (94%) patients receiving azithromycin, and 36 (100%) patients receiving ciprofloxacin (difference -6% [CI -14%–2%]). Peak serum concentrations of azithromycin were equal to the minimum inhibitory concentration (MIC) of the infecting shigella strains, whereas serum concentrations of ciprofloxacin were 28 times the MIC. Stool concentrations of both drugs were more than 200 times the MIC.

Treatment of Shigellosis: III. Comparison of One- or Two-dose Ciprofloxacin With Standard 5-Day Therapy. Treatment of Shigellosis: IV. Cefixime Is Ineffective in Shigellosis in Adults. Treatment of Shigellosis: V. Comparison of Azithromycin and Ciprofloxacin: A Double Blind, Randomized, Controlled Trial.

(continued)

Conclusion   A single 1-gram dose of ciprofloxacin is effective therapy for patients infected with species of shigella other than S. dysenteriae type 1. Single-dose therapy is inferior to 10-dose therapy for treating patients infected with S. dysenteriae type 1.

Cefixime is ineffective in treating shigellosis in adults when used in the standard recommended dosage.

Azithromycin is effective in the treatment of moderate to severe shigellosis caused by multi-drug resistant Shigella strains.

Randomised Comparison of Ciprofloxacin Suspension and Pivmecillinam for Childhood Shigellosis

Title	Randomised comparison of ciprofloxacin suspension and pivmecillinam for childhood shigellosis.
Authors	Salam MA, Dhar U, Khan WA, et al.
Reference	Lancet 1998;352:522–527.
Disease/ Pathogen	Shigellosis.
Purpose	To test the effects of ciprofloxacin treatment in children with shigella dysentery.
Design	Randomized, double blind.
Patients	143 children aged 2-15 years with dysentery of 72 h or less duration.
Follow-up	Patients stayed in hospital for 6 days, and were followed up 7, 30, and 180 days after hospital discharge. Joint symptoms and function were assessed daily for 6 days. Clinical success was defined as the absence of frank dysentery on day 3, and on day 5 no bloody-mucoid stools, one or no watery stool, six or fewer total stools, and no fever. If no shigella were isolated from fecal samples on day 3 or thereafter, treatment was judged bacteriologically successful.
Treatment/ prophylaxis regimen	Ciprofloxacin suspension (10 mg/kg every 12 h for 5 days, maximum individual dose 500 mg) or pivmecillinam tablets (15–20 mg/kg every 8 h for 5 days, maximum individual dose 300 mg).

(continued)

Results

13 patients were excluded since they did not meet eligibility criteria; 10 withdrew before day 5. Thus, 120 patients (60 in each group) completed the study. Treatment was clinically successful in 48 (80%) of 60 patients who received ciprofloxacin and in 39 (65%) of 60 patients who received pivmecillinam (p=0.1). Treatment was bacteriologically successful in all of the patients receiving ciprofloxacin, and in 54 (90%) of the patients receiving pivmecillinam (p=0.03). Joint pain after treatment began in 13 (18%) of 71 patients who received ciprofloxacin and 16 (22%) of 72 patients who received pivmecillinam (p>0.2), and no patient had signs of arthritis.

Conclusion

In this trial, ciprofloxacin suspension and pivmecillinam had the same clinical efficacy. Ciprofloxacin had greater bacteriological efficacy, and was not associated with the development of arthropathy. The authors conclude that ciprofloxacin is an effective and safe drug for use in multiply resistant childhood shigellosis.

2. Pathogens

nn. Staphylococcal Infections

Elimination of Coincident Staphylococcus Aureus Nasal and Hand Carriage with Intranasal Application of Mupirocin Calcium Ointment

Title	Elimination of coincident Staphylococcus aureus nasal and hand carriage with intranasal application of mupirocin calcium ointment.
Authors	Reagan DR, Doebbeling BN, Pfaller MA, et al.
Reference	Ann Intern Med 1991;114:101–106.
Disease/ Pathogen	Staphylococcus aureus carriage.
Purpose	To determine the safety and efficacy of mupirocin calcium ointment in the elimination of S. aureus nasal and hand carriage in healthy persons.
Design	A double blind, placebo controlled, randomized trial.
Patients	Health care workers with stable S. aureus nasal carriage.
Follow-up	Cultures of the hands and nares were obtained at baseline and 72 hours after therapy. The nares were also cultured 1, 2, 4, and 12 weeks after therapy. Antimicrobial susceptibility testing and restriction endonuclease analysis of plasmid DNA were used to confirm strain identity.
Treatment/ prophylaxis regimen	Subjects (n=68) were randomly assigned to receive either mupirocin or placebo intranasally twice daily for 5 days.

Elimination of Coincident Staphylococcus Aureus Nasal and Hand Carriage with Intranasal Application of Mupirocin Calcium Ointment

(continued)

Results
There were no serious side effects. Mupirocin decreased the frequency of S. aureus nasal carriage at each time interval: At 3 months, 71% of subjects receiving mupirocin remained free of nasal S. aureus, compared with 18% of controls. This difference (53%; 95% confidence interval [CI] 26%-80%) was significant (p<0.0001). Additionally, analysis of plasmid patterns showed that 79% of subjects in the mupirocin group were free of the initial colonizing strain at 3 months. The proportion of hand cultures positive for S. aureus in the mupirocin group after therapy was lower than in the placebo group (2.9%, compared with 57.6%). This difference (53%; 95 CI 30%-80%) was significant, after adjustment for the frequency of hand carriage at baseline (p<0.0001).

Conclusion
When applied intranasally for 5 days, mupirocin calcium ointment is safe and effective in eliminating S. aureus nasal carriage in healthy persons for up to 3 months and appears to have a corresponding effect on hand carriage at 72 hours after therapy.

Elimination of Staphylococcus Aureus Nasal Carriage
in Health Care Workers: Analysis of Six Clinical Trials
with Calcium Mupirocin Ointment.

Title	Elimination of Staphylococcus aureus nasal carriage in health care workers: Analysis of six clinical trials with calcium mupirocin ointment.
Authors	Doebbeling BN, Breneman DL, Neu HC, et al.
Reference	Clin Infect Dis 1993;17(3):466–474.
Disease/ Pathogen	Staphylococcus aureus infections.
Purpose	To evaluate the efficacy and safety of calcium mupirocin ointment in eliminating nasal carriage of S. aureus among health care workers.
Design	Randomized, double blind, multicenter.
Patients	Healthy volunteers with stable nasal carriage of S. aureus (n=339).
Follow-up	5 days.
Treatment/ prophylaxis regimen	Patients received either calcium mupirocin ointment (n=170) or an identical placebo ointment (n=169) intranasally for 5 days.

Elimination of Staphylococcus Aureus Nasal Carriage in Health Care Workers: Analysis of Six Clinical Trials with Calcium Mupirocin Ointment.

(continued)

Results

Nasal carriage was eliminated 48-96 hours after completion of treatment in 130 (91%) of 143 evaluable volunteers receiving mupirocin, but in only eight (6%) of 142 evaluable volunteers receiving placebo. The 85% crude difference represents a 90% pooled (adjusted) estimate of the risk difference (95% confidence interval [CI] 0.86–0.95) and a risk ratio of 16 ($p < 0.0001$). This effect of treatment with mupirocin was observed consistently (risk ratio 8–32) in all six centers. In addition, 96 of the 130 mupirocin-treated volunteers and one of the eight placebo-treated volunteers who were culture-negative at the end of therapy remained free of S. aureus 4 weeks after treatment. Adverse events in each treatment arm were mild and equally frequent.

Conclusion

These data, consistent across six institutions, demonstrate that calcium mupirocin ointment administered intranasally for 5 days is safe and effective in eliminating stable nasal carriage of S. aureus.

2. Pathogens

oo. Streptococcal Infections

Role of Benzathine Penicillin G in Prophylaxis for Recurrent Streptococcal Cellulitis of the Lower Legs

Title	Role of benzathine penicillin G in prophylaxis for recurrent streptococcal cellulitis of the lower legs.
Authors	Wang JH, Liu YC, Cheng DL, et al.
Reference	Clin Infect Dis 1997;25(3):685–689.
Disease/ Pathogen	Streptococcal infections.
Purpose	To evaluate the use of monthly intramuscular injections of benzathine penicillin G to prevent recurrences of cellulitis.
Design	Prospective study.
Patients	A total of 115 patients with definite or presumptive cases of streptococcal cellulitis were enrolled in this study. 84 of these patients who declined follow-up or received incomplete prophylaxis were considered controls.
Follow-up	Recurrence of cellulitis.
Treatment/ prophylaxis regimen	31 individuals received prophylaxis with intramuscular injections of benzathin penicillin G and controls did not receive prophylaxis.

(continued)

Results   Recurrence occurred in four (12.9%) of 31 cases who received prophylaxis and 16 (19%) of the 84 cases who did not receive prophylaxis. The difference was not statistically significant. Predisposing factors for cellulitis were found in 57 (49.6%) of the 115 enrolled cases, and were mostly related to the impairment of local circulation. Administration of prophylaxis successfully reduced the recurrence rate to zero among patients without predisposing factors but failed to prevent recurrence in those with predisposing factors (20%).

Conclusion   The authors conclude that monthly benzathine penicillin G prophylaxis benefits only patients without predisposing factors for cellulitis.

Evaluation of Short-Course Therapy with Cefixime or Rifampin for Eradication of Pharyngeally Carried Group A Streptococci

Title	Evaluation of short-course therapy with cefixime or rifampin for eradication of pharyngeally carried group A streptococci.
Authors	Davies HD, Low DE, Schwartz B, et al.
Reference	Clin Infect Dis 1995;21(5):1294–1299.
Disease/ Pathogen	Group A streptococci.
Purpose	To evaluate short course with cefixime or rifampin for the treatment of pharyngeally carried group A streptococci (GAS).
Design	Randomized, controlled trial.
Patients	131 contacts of patients with GAS infections who were screened for pharyngeal GAS colonization and were positive.
Treatment/ prophylaxis regimen	Patients were randomized to receive either cefixime (8 mg/[kg.d]; maximum 400 mg) or rifampin (20 mg/kg; maximum, 600 mg) once a day for 4 days.

Evaluation of Short-Course Therapy with Cefixime or Rifampin for Eradication of Pharyngeally Carried Group A Streptococci

(continued)

Results	2 to 5 days following completion of therapy, repeated cultures were negative for 13 (38%) of 34 rifampin recipients, and 71 (77%; 95% confidence interval [CI] 69%–85%) of 97 cefixime recipients. At 10-14 days after treatment, only 53% of cefixime recipients remained culture-negative. Rates of successful clearance improved with increasing age (p<0.01); among 17 adults who received cefixime, the success rate was 94%.
Conclusion	4 days of therapy with rifampin is not effective for eradication of pharyngeally carried GAS. 4 days of therapy with cefixime may be effective for adults, but further studies are needed.

2. Pathogens

pp. Strongyloidiasis

A Randomized Trial of Single- and Two-Dose Ivermectin Vs Thiabendazole for Treatment of Strongyloidiasis

Title	A randomized trial of single- and two-dose ivermectin vs thiabendazole for treatment of strongyloidiasis.
Authors	Gann PH, Neva FA, Gam AA.
Reference	J Infect Dis 1994;169(5):1076–1079.
Disease/ Pathogen	Strongyloidiasis.
Purpose	To compare ivermectin and thiabendazole for treatment of chronic infection with Strongyloides stercoralis.
Design	Randomized trial
Patients	Patients infected with S. stercoralis.
Follow-up	Stools were examined 7 days and 1, 3, 6, 10, and 22 months after treatment.
Treatment/ prophylaxis regimen	Subjects received ivermectin (200 micrograms/kg) in a single dose, ivermectin (200 micrograms/kg) on two consecutive days, or thiabendazole (50 mg/kg/day) twice daily for three consecutive days.

(continued)

Results

Most subjects (94%) had intermittent symptoms, including urticaria, epigastric pain, and diarrhea. 53 subjects completed at least 3 months of follow-up. Only one of 34 and two of 19 ivermectin and thiabendazole subjects, respectively, had a stool positive for larvae after treatment. Symptoms were relieved in all three groups and eosinophil levels returned to normal in 90% of all subjects by 12 months. Nearly 95% of thiabendazole subjects had short-term adverse effects during therapy vs only 18% of those treated with ivermectin.

Conclusion

One dose of ivermectin provides safety and efficacy equivalent to thiabendazole with a much lower prevalence of side effects and, consequently, better compliance.

2. Pathogens

qq. Toxoplasmosis

Early and Longitudinal Evaluations of Treated Infants and Children and Untreated Historical Patients with Congenital Toxoplasmosis

Title	Early and longitudinal evaluations of treated infants and children and untreated historical patients with congenital toxoplasmosis.
Authors	McAuley J, Boyer KM, Patel D, et al.
Reference	Clin Infect Dis 1994;18(1):38–72.
Disease/Pathogen	Toxoplasmosis.
Purpose	To compare the early and longitudinal evaluations of infants and children who were treated for congenital toxoplasmosis with those who were untreated.
Design	Uniform evaluation and case history.
Patients	44 infants and children with congenital toxoplasmosis.
Follow-up	10 years.

***Early and Longitudinal Evaluations of Treated Infants
and Children and Untreated Historical Patients with
Congenital Toxoplasmosis***

(continued)

Results

Factors that contributed to the more severe disabilities included delayed diagnosis and initiation of therapy; prolonged, concomitant neonatal hypoxia and hypoglycemia; profound visual impairment; and prolonged, uncorrected increased intracranial pressure with hydrocephalus and compression of the brain. Years after therapy was discontinued, three children developed new retinal lesions (without loss of visual acuity when therapy for Toxoplasma gondii was initiated promptly), and three children experienced a new onset of afebrile seizures. Most remarkable were the normal developmental, neurological, and ophthalmologic findings at the early follow-up evaluations of many—but not all—of the treated children, despite severe manifestations, such as substantial systemic disease, hydrocephalus, microcephalus, multiple intracranial calcifications, and extensive macular destruction detected at birth.

Conclusion

These favorable outcomes contrast markedly with outcomes reported previously for children with congenital toxoplasmosis who were untreated or treated for only 1 month.

2. Pathogens
rr. Traveler's Diarrhea

Treatment of Traveler's Diarrhea: Ciprofloxacin Plus Loperamide Compared with Ciprofloxacin Alone: A Placebo Controlled, Randomized Trial.

Title	Treatment of traveler's diarrhea: Ciprofloxacin plus loperamide compared with ciprofloxacin alone: A placebo controlled, randomized trial.
Authors	Taylor DN, Sanchez JL, Candler W, et al.
Reference	Ann Intern Med 1991;114:731–734.
Disease/ Pathogen	Traveler's diarrhea.
Purpose	To compare the safety and efficacy of loperamide used in combination with ciprofloxacin or ciprofloxacin alone for the treatment of traveler's diarrhea.
Design	Double blind, placebo controlled, randomized, clinical trial.
Patients	United States military personnel with traveler's diarrhea (n=104). Persons who were noncompliant, had bloody diarrhea, or had received antidiarrheal medications before entry into the study were excluded.
Follow-up	Enterotoxigenic Escherichia coli was isolated from 57% of patients; shigella and salmonella, seen in 4% and 2% of patients, respectively, were not common.

Treatment of Traveler's Diarrhea: Ciprofloxacin Plus Loperamide Compared with Ciprofloxacin Alone: A Placebo Controlled, Randomized Trial.

(continued)

Treatment/ prophylaxis regimen	All participants with traveler's diarrhea were treated with ciprofloxacin, 500 mg twice daily for 3 days. 50 of these patients were randomly assigned to receive loperamide, a 4-mg first dose, and 2 mg for every loose stool (as much as 16 mg/d), and 54 were randomly assigned to receive placebo.
Results	After 24 hours, the symptoms of 82% of patients in the ciprofloxacin and loperamide group, compared with 67% in the ciprofloxacin and placebo group had improved or fully recovered (odds ratio 2.3; 95% confidence interval [CI] 0.8–6.3; p=0.08). After 48 hours, the symptoms of 90% of both groups had improved or fully recovered. The mean number of stools for those receiving loperamide was not much lower than those who did not receive loperamide after 24 hours (1.9±0.2 [SE], compared with 2.6±0.2) or 48 hours (3.1±0.3, compared with 4.0±0.3) of treatment (p=0.19).
Conclusion	In a region where enterotoxigenic E. coli was the predominant cause of traveler's diarrhea, loperamide combined with ciprofloxacin was not better than treatment with ciprofloxacin alone. Loperamide appeared to have some benefit in the first 24 hours of treatment in patients infected with enterotoxigenic E. coli. Both regimens were safe.

Randomised Trial of Single-Dose Ciprofloxacin for Traveler's Diarrhea

Title	Randomised trial of single-dose ciprofloxacin for traveler's diarrhea.
Authors	Salam I, Katelaris P, Leigh-Smith S, et al.
Reference	Lancet 1994;344:1537–1539.
Disease/ Pathogen	Traveler's diarrhea.
Purpose	To compare the efficacy of a single 500 mg dose of ciprofloxacin with placebo for treatment of acute diarrhea in travelers.
Design	Randomized, placebo controlled trial.
Patients	British troops who were within their first 8 weeks of deployment in Belize and who presented within 24 h of the onset of diarrhea. 88 subjects enrolled, 83 were evaluable, of whom 45 received ciprofloxacin, and 38 placebo.
Follow-up	Every subject recorded the number and consistency of stools and presence of any other associated symptoms for 72 h or until recovery.
Treatment/ prophylaxis regimen	Patients were randomized to receive either ciprofloxacin 500 mg or placebo.

Results

Groups did not differ with regard to duration or severity of diarrhea at randomisation. Mean (SE) duration of diarrhea, as assessed by time to the last liquid and last unformed stool, was reduced from 50.4 (4.5) h and 53.5 (4.4) h, respectively, in the placebo group to 20.9 (3.4) h and 24.8 (3.8) h in those receiving ciprofloxacin (p<0.0001). Mean number of liquid stools was reduced from 11.4 (1.2) in the placebo group to 5 (0.7) in the ciprofloxacin-treated group (p < 0.0001). The cumulative percentages of subjects with no unformed stool after 24 h, 48 h, and 72 h were, respectively, 64%, 82%, and 93% in the ciprofloxacin group and 11%, 42%, and 79% in the placebo group (p<0.0001, p<0.001, and not significant, respectively).

Conclusion

A single 500 mg dose of ciprofloxacin was an effective empirical treatment for reducing the duration and severity of diarrhea in travelers. The regimen should maximise compliance and reduce the cost and duration of therapy.

Title	Treatment of traveler's diarrhea with sulfamethoxazole and trimethoprim and loperamide.
Authors	Ericsson CD, DuPont HL, Mathewson JJ, et al.
Reference	JAMA 1990;263(2):257–261.
Disease/ Pathogen	Traveler's diarrhea.
Purpose	To determine the efficacy of sulfamethoxazole and trimethoprim and loperamide for the treatment of traveler's diarrhea.
Design	Randomized, double blind, placebo controlled trial
Patients	227 U.S. adults with acute diarrhea in Mexico.
Treatment/ prophylaxis regimen	Patients received a single dose of sulfamethoxazole and trimethoprim (1600/320 mg) or 3 days of therapy with loperamide hydrochloride (4-mg loading dose, then 2 mg orally after each loose stool), sulfamethoxazole-trimethoprim (800/160 mg orally twice daily), or the combination of both.

Results	Subjects treated with the combination had the shortest average duration of diarrhea, compared with the placebo group (1 hour vs 59 hours), took the least amount of loperamide after the loading dose (3.8 mg), and had the shortest duration of diarrhea associated with fecal leukocytes or blood-tinged stools (4.5 hours). A single dose of sulfamethoxazole-trimethoprim was also efficacious (28 vs 59 hours), but loperamide alone was significantly effective only when treatment failures were treated with antibiotics (33 vs 58 hours).
Conclusion	The combination of sulfamethoxazole-trimethoprim plus loperamide can be highly recommended for the treatment of most patients with traveler's diarrhea.

Treatment of Traveler's Diarrhea with Ciprofloxacin and Loperamide

Title	Treatment of traveler's diarrhea with ciprofloxacin and loperamide.
Authors	Petruccelli BP, Murphy GS, Sanchez JL, et al.
Reference	J Infect Dis 1992;165(3):557–560.
Disease/ Pathogen	Traveler's diarrhea.
Purpose	To determine the efficacy of loperamide given with long- and short-course quinolone therapy for treating traveler's diarrhea.
Design	Randomized, clinical trial.
Patients	142 U.S. military personnel.
Treatment/ prophylaxis regimen	Patients received a single 750-mg dose of ciprofloxacin with placebo, 750 mg of ciprofloxacin with loperamide, or a 3-day course of 500 mg of ciprofloxacin twice daily with loperamide

Treatment of Traveler's Diarrhea with Ciprofloxacin and Loperamide

(continued)

Results	Culture of pretreatment stool specimens revealed campylobacters (41%), salmonellae (18%), enterotoxigenic Escherichia coli (ETEC, 6%), and shigellae (4%). Of the participants, 87% completely recovered within 72 h of entry. Total duration of illness did not differ significantly among the three treatment groups, but patients in the 3-day ciprofloxacin plus loperamide group reported a lower cumulative number of liquid bowel movements at 48 and 72 h after enrollment compared with patients in the single-dose ciprofloxacin plus placebo group (1.8 vs 3.6, $p=0.01$; 2 vs 3.9, $p=0.01$).
Conclusion	While not delivering a remarkable therapeutic advantage, loperamide appears to be safe for treatment of non-ETEC causes of traveler's diarrhea. Two of 54 patients with Campylobacter enteritis had a clinical relapse after treatment that was associated with development of ciprofloxacin resistance.

2. Pathogens

ss. Trichomoniasis

Title	A double blind, placebo controlled trial of single-dose intravaginal vs single-dose oral metronidazole in the treatment of trichomonal vaginitis.
Authors	Tidwell BH, Lushbaugh WB, Laughlin MD, et al.
Reference	J Infect Dis 1994;170(1):242–246.
Disease/ Pathogen	Trichomonas infections.
Purpose	To compare single dose intravaginal vs single dose oral metronidazole in the treatment of trichomonal vaginitis.
Design	Randomized, double blind, placebo controlled trial.
Patients	Patients with a culture positive for trichomonas organisms.
Treatment/ prophylaxis regimen	Patients were given either a single 2-g intravaginal dose of metronidazole cream or a single 2-g oral dose of metronidazole

(continued)

Results

Of the 302 pre-enrollment cultures completed, 94 (31%) were positive. 61 patients were enrolled in the study. Each received either oral placebo and intravaginal metronidazole or intravaginal placebo and oral metronidazole. Follow-up cultures were done on post-treatment day 3-5. Of the 53 evaluatable patients, 14 (50%) of 28 in the intravaginal group and 22 (88%) of 25 in the oral group were microbiologically cured ($p=0.0037$).

Conclusion

Single-dose intravaginal metronidazole is inferior to single-dose oral metronidazole and cannot be relied on as an alternative therapy.

2. Pathogens

tt. Tuberculosis

Randomised, Controlled Trial of Self-Supervised and Directly Observed Treatment of Tuberculosis

Title	Randomised, controlled trial of self-supervised and directly observed treatment of tuberculosis.
Authors	Zwarenstein M, Schoeman JH, Vundule C, et al.
Reference	Lancet 1998;352:1340–1343.
Disease/ Pathogen	Tuberculosis.
Purpose	To compare direct observation (DO) with self-supervision, in which patients on the same drug regimen are not observed taking their pills, to assess the effect of each on the success of tuberculosis treatment.
Design	Unblinded, randomised, controlled trial in two communities with large tuberculosis caseloads.
Patients	The trial included 216 adults who started pulmonary tuberculosis treatment for the first time, or who had a second course of treatment (retreatment patients).
Follow-up	Analysis was by intention to treat. Individual patient data from the two communities were combined.
Treatment/ prophylaxis regimen	Direct observation with self-supervision, in which patients on the same drug regimen are not observed taking their pills.

(continued)

Results   Treatment for tuberculosis was more successful among self-supervised patients (60% of patients) than among those on DO (54% of patients, difference between groups 6% [90% confidence interval [CI] -5.1–17]). Retreatment patients had significantly more successful treatment outcomes if self-supervised (74% of patients) than on DO (42% of patients, difference between groups 32% [11%–52%]).

Conclusion   At high rates of treatment interruption, self-supervision achieved equivalent outcomes to clinic DO at lower cost. Self-supervision achieved better outcomes for retreatment patients. Supportive patient-carer relations, rather than the authoritarian surveillance implicit in DO, may improve treatment outcomes and help to control tuberculosis.

3. Infections in Special Hosts

a. Infections in Immunocompromised Patients

High-Dose Weekly Intravenous Immunoglobulin to Prevent Infections in Patients Undergoing Autologous Bone Marrow Transplantation or Severe Myelosuppressive Therapy: A Study of the American Bone Marrow Transplant Group.

Title	High-dose weekly intravenous immunoglobulin to prevent infections in patients undergoing autologous bone marrow transplantation or severe myelosuppressive therapy: A Study of the American Bone Marrow Transplant Group.
Authors	Wolff SN, Fay JW, Herzig RH, et al.
Reference	Ann Intern Med 1993;118:937–942.
Disease/ Pathogen	Systemic infections.
Purpose	To determine whether intravenous immunoglobulin (IVIG) prevents severe infections during autologous bone marrow transplantation or equivalent high-dose myelosuppressive therapy.
Design	Randomized, stratified, nonblinded study.
Patients	170 patients entered the study; 82 received IVIG and 88 were untreated controls. The study groups were similar for parameters capable of influencing the likelihood of infection.
Follow-up	The development of bloodstream or other clinically proven infection, platelet use, and the development of alloimmunity to platelet transfusion.

***High-Dose Weekly Intravenous Immunoglobulin to Prevent
Infections in Patients Undergoing Autologous Bone Marrow
Transplantation or Severe Myelosuppressive Therapy:
A Study of the American Bone Marrow Transplant Group.***

(continued)

Treatment/ prophylaxis regimen	IVIG was given weekly at a dose of 500 mg/kg body weight from the initiation of cytotoxic therapy to the resolution of neutropenia.
Results	Clinical infection, bacteremia, and fungemia occurred in 43%, 35%, and 6% of the IVIG-treated patients, and in 44%, 34%, and 9% of the control patients. Gram-positive bacteremia and gram-negative bacteremia occurred in 28% and 11% of the IVIG group, and in 23% and 13% of the control group. Death due to infection occurred in 4.9% of IVIG recipients, and in 2.3% of controls. None of these observations was statistically significant (p>0.2). Survival to hospital discharge was achieved in 86.6% of the IVIG group, and in 96.6% of the control group. The survival difference (10%; 95% confidence interval [CI] 1.7%–18.3%; p=0.02) was due to a higher incidence of regimen-related toxic death in the IVIG-treated group.
Conclusion	The use of IVIG did not prevent infection. Fewer deaths occurred among controls due to a higher incidence of fatal hepatic veno-occlusive disease in patients receiving IVIG.

Prevention of Bacterial Infection in Neutropenic Patients with Hematologic Malignancies: A Randomized, Multicenter Trial Comparing Norfloxacin with Ciprofloxacin.

Title	Prevention of bacterial infection in neutropenic patients with hematologic malignancies: A randomized, multicenter trial comparing norfloxacin with ciprofloxacin.
Reference	Ann Intern Med 1991;115:7–12.
Disease/ Pathogen	Bacterial infections.
Purpose	To compare the efficacy of norfloxacin and ciprofloxacin in preventing bacterial infection in neutropenic patients.
Design	A randomized, controlled, multicenter trial.
Patients	801 consecutive, afebrile, adult patients who had hematologic malignancies, or who had bone marrow transplantation and chemotherapy-induced neutropenia (neutrophil count, less than 1000/mm³) expected to last more than 10 days.
Follow-up	Efficacy analysis was done for 619 patients: 319 treated with norfloxacin and 300 treated with ciprofloxacin.
Treatment/ prophylaxis regimen	Patients were randomly assigned to receive orally every 12 hours norfloxacin, 400 mg, or ciprofloxacin, 500 mg.

Prevention of Bacterial Infection in Neutropenic Patients with Hematologic Malignancies: A Randomized, Multicenter Trial Comparing Norfloxacin with Ciprofloxacin.

(continued)

Results   More patients receiving ciprofloxacin did not develop fever during neutropenia and did not receive antibiotics (34%), compared with those receiving norfloxacin (25%) (p=0.01). Patients receiving ciprofloxacin had a lower rate of microbiologically documented infection (17%, compared with 24%; p=0.058), particularly of infection from gram-negative bacilli (4%, compared with 9%; p=0.03). The interval to the first febrile episode was also longer in patients receiving ciprofloxacin (8.3, compared with 7.2 days; p=0.055). The rates of clinically documented infection, fever of unknown origin, and mortality, as well as compliance and tolerability, were similar in the two groups. Patients who had neutropenia for less than 15 days, who had severe neutropenia for less than 7 days, and who received antifungal prophylaxis benefited most from ciprofloxacin therapy.

Conclusion   Ciprofloxacin should be used to prevent the development of infection in neutropenic patients with hematologic malignancies.

Fluconazole Prophylaxis of Fungal Infections in Patients with Acute Leukemia: Results of a Randomized Placebo Controlled, Double Blind, Multicenter Trial.

Title	Fluconazole prophylaxis of fungal infections in patients with acute leukemia: Results of a randomized placebo controlled, double blind, multicenter trial.
Authors	Winston DJ, Chandrasekar PH, Lazarus HM, et al.
Reference	Ann Intern Med 1993;118:495–503.
Disease/ Pathogen	Infections among immunosupressed patients.
Purpose	To evaluate the efficacy and safety of fluconazole for prevention of fungal infections.
Design	A randomized, placebo controlled, double blind, multicenter trial.
Patients	Adults (257) undergoing chemotherapy for acute leukemia.
Follow-up	Fungal colonization, proven superficial or invasive fungal infection, empiric antifungal therapy with amphotericin B, drug-related side effects, and mortality.
Treatment/ prophylaxis regimen	Patients were randomly assigned to receive either fluconazole (400 mg orally once daily or 200 mg intravenously every 12 hours) or placebo. The study drug was started at initiation of chemotherapy and continued until recovery of neutrophil count, development of proven or suspected invasive fungal infection, or the occurrence of a drug-related toxicity.

Fluconazole Prophylaxis of Fungal Infections in Patients with Acute Leukemia: Results of a Randomized Placebo Controlled, Double Blind, Multicenter Trial.

(continued)

Results   Fluconazole decreased fungal colonization in 83 of 122 (68%) placebo patients, compared with 34 of 119 (29%) fluconazole patients colonized at end of prophylaxis, (p<0.001) and proven fungal infections in 27 of 132 (21%) placebo patients, compared with 11 of 123 (9%) fluconazole patients infected (p=0.02). Superficial fungal infections occurred in 20 of 132 (15%) placebo patients but in only 7 of 123 (6%) fluconazole patients (p= 0.01), whereas invasive fungal infections developed in 10 of 132 (8%) placebo patients and in 5 of 123 (4%) fluconazole patients (p=0.3). Fluconazole was especially effective in eliminating colonization and infection by candida species, other than Candida krusei in 66 of 122 (64%) placebo patients colonized at end of prophylaxis, compared with 11 of 119 (9%) fluconazole patients, (p<0.001; 22 of 132 (17%) placebo patients infected, compared with 7 of 123 (6%) fluconazole patients, (p=0.005). Aspergillus infections were infrequent in both fluconazole (three cases) and placebo groups (three cases). The use of amphotericin B, the incidence of drug-related side effects, and overall mortality, were similar in both study groups.

Conclusion   Prophylactic fluconazole prevents colonization and superficial infections by candida species other than Candida krusei in patients undergoing chemotherapy for acute leukemia, and is well tolerated. Fluconazole could not be clearly shown to be effective for preventing invasive fungal infections, reducing the use of amphotericin B, or decreasing the number of deaths.

A Controlled Trial of Fluconazole to Prevent Fungal Infections in Patients Undergoing Bone Marrow Transplantation

Title	A controlled trial of fluconazole to prevent fungal infections in patients undergoing bone marrow transplantation.
Authors	Goodman JL, Winston DJ, Greenfield RA, et al.
Reference	N Engl J Med 1992;326:845–851.
Disease/ Pathogen	Fungal infections.
Purpose	To determine the effectiveness of fluconazole in preventing fungal infections in patients undergoing bone marrow transplantation.
Design	Randomized, double blind, multicenter.
Patients	Patients receiving bone marrow transplants
Follow-up	Until the neutrophil count returned to 1000 per microliter, toxicity was suspected, or a systemic fungal infection, was suspected or proved.
Treatment/ prophylaxis regimen	Placebo or fluconazole (400 mg daily prophylactically from the start of the conditioning regimen).

A Controlled Trial of Fluconazole to Prevent Fungal Infections in Patients Undergoing Bone Marrow Transplantation

(continued)

Results

By the end of the treatment period, 67.2% of the 177 patients assigned to placebo had a positive fungal culture of specimens from any site, as compared with 29.6% of the 179 patients assigned to fluconazole. Among these, superficial infections were diagnosed in 33.3% of the patients receiving placebo, and in 8.4% of the patients receiving fluconazole (p<0.001). Systemic fungal infections occurred in 28 patients who received placebo, as compared with five who received fluconazole (15.8% vs 2.8%, p<0.001). Fluconazole prevented infection with all strains of candida except Candida krusei. Fluconazole was well tolerated, although patients who received it had a higher mean increase in alanine aminotransferase levels than patients who received placebo. Although there was no significant difference in overall mortality between the groups, fewer deaths were ascribed to acute systemic fungal infections in the group receiving fluconazole than in the group receiving placebo (one of 179 vs 10 of 177, p<0.001).

Conclusion

Prophylactic administration of fluconazole to recipients of bone marrow transplants reduces the incidence of both systemic and superficial fungal infections.

Quinolone-Based Antibacterial Chemoprophylaxis in Neutropenic Patients: Effect of Augmented Gram-Positive Activity on Infectious Morbidity.

Title	Quinolone-based antibacterial chemoprophylaxis in neutropenic patients: Effect of augmented gram-positive activity on infectious morbidity.
Authors	Bow EJ, Mandell LA, Louie TJ, et al
Reference	Ann Intern Med 1996;125:183–190.
Disease/ Pathogen	Infections among immunocompromised patients.
Purpose	To determine whether augmented quinolone-based antibacterial prophylaxis in neutropenic patients with cancer reduces infections caused by gram-positive cocci and preserves the protective effect against aerobic gram-negative bacilli.
Design	Open, randomized, controlled, multicenter, clinical trial.
Patients	111 eligible and evaluable patients hospitalized for severe neutropenia (neutrophil count $<0.5 \times 10^9$/L lasting at least 14 days) who were receiving cytotoxic therapy for acute leukemia or bone marrow autografting.
Follow-up	Incidence and cause of suspected or proven infection.
Treatment/ prophylaxis regimen	One of three oral antibacterial prophylactic regimens (norfloxacin, 400 mg every 12 hours; ofloxacin, 400 mg every 12 hours; or ofloxacin, 400 mg, plus rifampin, 300 mg, every 12 hours) beginning with cytotoxic therapy.

Quinolone-Based Antibacterial Chemoprophylaxis in Neutropenic Patients: Effect of Augmented Gram-Positive Activity on Infectious Morbidity.

(continued)

Results

Microbiologically documented overall infection rates for norfloxacin, ofloxacin, and ofloxacin plus rifampin were 47%, 24%, and 9%, respectively (p<0.001). Corresponding rates were 24%, 13%, and 3%, respectively, for staphylococcal bacteremia (p=0.03), and 21%, 3%, and 3%, respectively, for streptococcal bacteremia (p<0.01). The pattern of bacteremia suggested that rifampin played a role in suppressing staphylococcal infection. Both ofloxacin alone, and ofloxacin plus rifampin, had a clinically significant antistreptococcal effect. Aerobic gram-negative rods were cleared from rectal surveillance cultures in all patients after a median of 5.5 days and caused infection in only one patient (0.9%). The reductions in the number of microbiologically documented infections among ofloxacin recipients and ofloxacin plus rifampin recipients were offset by concomitant increases in the number of unexplained fevers (24% of norfloxacin recipients, 53% of ofloxacin recipients, and 49% of ofloxacin plus rifampin recipients; p=0.02). No statistically significant differences were found among the treatment arms, with respect to the overall incidence of febrile neutropenic episodes as defined for this trial (79% for the norfloxacin group, 82% for the ofloxacin group, and 77% for the ofloxacin plus rifampin group).

Conclusion

Quinolone-based antibacterial chemoprophylaxis protected patients from aerobic gram-negative bacillary infections. Augmentation of the gram-positive activity reduced the incidence of gram-positive infections but did not influence the overall incidence of febrile neutropenic episodes.

Preventing Fungal Infection in Neutropenic Patients with Acute Leukemia: Fluconazole Compared with Oral Amphotericin B.

Title	Preventing fungal infection in neutropenic patients with acute leukemia: Fluconazole compared with oral amphotericin B.
Authors	Menichett F, Del Favero A, Martino P, et al.
Reference	Ann Intern Med 1994;120:913–918.
Disease/ Pathogen	Systemic fungal infection.
Purpose	To compare the efficacy and tolerability of fluconazole and oral amphotericin B in preventing fungal infection in neutropenic patients with acute leukemia.
Design	A randomized, controlled, multicenter trial.
Patients	820 consecutive, afebrile, adult patients with acute leukemia and chemotherapy-induced neutropenia.
Treatment/ prophylaxis regimen	Patients were randomly assigned to receive fluconazole, 150 mg, as a once-daily capsule, or amphotericin B suspension, 500 mg every 6 hours.

Preventing Fungal Infection in Neutropenic Patients with Acute Leukemia: Fluconazole Compared with Oral Amphotericin B.

(continued)

Results
Definite systemic fungal infection occurred in 2.6% of fluconazole recipients, and 2.5% of amphotericin B recipients; suspected systemic fungal infection requiring the empiric use of intravenous amphotericin B occurred in 16% of fluconazole recipients, and 21% of oral amphotericin B recipients, a difference of 5 percentage points (95% confidence interval [CI] for difference -0.02%-10%; p=0.07). Superficial fungal infection was documented in 1.7% of fluconazole recipients, compared with 2.7% of amphotericin B recipients, a difference of 1 percentage point (CI of differences -0.9%-3%; p>0.2). The distribution of fungal isolates in systemic and superficial fungal infection was similar in both groups. The overall mortality rate accounted for 10% in both groups. An excellent compliance was documented for 90% of patients treated with fluconazole, compared with 72% of those treated with amphotericin B suspension, a difference of 18 percentage points (CI for difference 13%-23%). Side-effects were documented less frequently in fluconazole than in amphotericin B recipients (1.4%, compared with 7%, a difference of 5.6 percentage points; CI for difference 2%-8%; p<0.01).

Conclusion
Fluconazole was at least as effective as oral amphotericin B in preventing systemic and superficial fungal infection, and the empiric use of amphotericin B in neutropenic patients with acute leukemia but was better tolerated.

Efficacy and Toxicity of Single Daily Doses of Amikacin and Ceftriaxone Vs Multiple Daily Doses of Amikacin and Ceftazidime for Infection in Patients with Cancer and Granulocytopenia

Title	Efficacy and toxicity of single daily doses of amikacin and ceftriaxone vs multiple daily doses of amikacin and ceftazidime for infection in patients with cancer and granulocytopenia.
Reference	Ann Intern Med 1993;119:584–593.
Disease/ Pathogen	Infections among immunocompromised patients.
Purpose	To compare the efficacy and toxicity of single daily dosing of amikacin and ceftriaxone with that of multiple daily dosing of amikacin and ceftazidime for febrile episodes in patients with cancer and granulocytopenia.
Design	A prospective, randomized, unblinded, multicenter trial.
Patients	677 patients with cancer and granulocytopenia (858 febrile episodes).
Treatment/ prophylaxis regimen	Random assignment to empiric therapy with a single daily dose of amikacin (20 mg/kg) and ceftriaxone (adults, 30 mg/kg; children, 80 mg/kg) (24-hour group) or with multiple daily doses of amikacin (6.5 mg/kg every 8 hours) and ceftazidime (33 mg/kg every 8 hours) (8-hour group).

Efficacy and Toxicity of Single Daily Doses of Amikacin and Ceftriaxone Vs Multiple Daily Doses of Amikacin and Ceftazidime for Infection in Patients with Cancer and Granulocytopenia

(continued)

Results   Single daily dosing of amikacin and ceftriaxone was as effective as multiple daily dosing of amikacin and ceftazidime (71%, compared with 74%; difference -3%; 95% confidence interval [CI] -10%–3%; p>0.2). Equivalent responses also were noted for each category of infection. Median peak (30 minutes after a 60-minute infusion) serum concentrations of amikacin were higher in the 24-hour group than in the 8-hour group (45.6, compared with 21 micrograms/mL, p<0.001), whereas trough (pre-infusion) levels were lower (0.9, compared with 2 micrograms/mL, p<0.001). Nephrotoxicity was 3% in the 24-hour group and 2% in the 8-hour group (difference, 1%; CI -1%–4%). Increases in serum creatinine, however, were delayed (p=0.048) and smaller (p=0.06) in the 24-hour group than in the 8-hour group, and occurred almost exclusively after other nephrotoxic drugs were added. Audiometry was only done in 144 patients (21%). Ototoxicity was 9% in the 24-hour group, and 7% in the 8-hour group (difference 2%; CI -7%–11%; p>0.2). Further infections developed in 15% and 12% of patients, respectively (difference 3%; CI -2%–9%). The overall mortality rate was 11% in both treatment groups (difference 0%; CI 5%–5%).

Conclusion   Single daily dosing of amikacin and ceftriaxone was as effective and no more toxic than multiple daily dosing of amikacin and ceftazidime for the empiric therapy of infection in patients with cancer and granulocytopenia.

Beta-Lactam Antibiotic Therapy in Febrile Granulocytopenic Patients: A Randomized Trial Comparing Cefoperazone Plus Piperacillin, Ceftazidime Plus Piperacillin, and Imipenem Alone.

Title	Beta-lactam antibiotic therapy in febrile granulocytopenic patients: A randomized trial comparing cefoperazone plus piperacillin, ceftazidime plus piperacillin, and imipenem alone.
Authors	Winston DJ, Ho WG, Bruckner DA, et al.
Reference	Ann Intern Med 1991;115:849–859.
Disease/ Pathogen	Infections among immunocompromised patients.
Purpose	To compare the efficacy, toxicity, and cost-effectiveness of double beta-lactam therapy with monotherapy.
Design	A randomized, controlled trial.
Patients	Febrile, granulocytopenic patients (429).
Follow-up	Clinical improvement, eradication of the infecting organism, and toxicity in 403 evaluable patients with one or more infections.
Treatment/ prophylaxis regimen	Patients were randomly assigned to receive IV cefoperazone (3 g every 12 hours) plus piperacillin (75 mg/kg body weight every 6 hours), ceftazidime (2 g every 8 hours) plus piperacillin (75 mg/kg every 6 hours), or imipenem alone (1 g or 0.5 g every 6 hours). Patients also received prophylactic vitamin K.

Beta-Lactam Antibiotic Therapy in Febrile Granulocytopenic Patients: A Randomized Trial Comparing Cefoperazone Plus Piperacillin, Ceftazidime Plus Piperacillin, and Imipenem Alone.

(continued)

Results

Cefoperazone and ceftazidime, when given in combination with piperacillin, were equally effective (response rates of 75% (104 of 138 patients) and 74% (101 of 137 patients), respectively. Monotherapy with imipenem had a response rate of 82% (111 of 136 patients), and was as effective as double beta-lactam therapy. Overall, antibiotic-related toxicity was minimal, although seizures were associated with high doses of imipenem. Seizures occurred in three of 29 patients (10.3%) who were receiving 4 g/d of imipenem, in three of 136 patients (2.2%) who were receiving cefoperazone plus piperacillin, in 0 of the 132 patients who were receiving ceftazidime plus piperacillin, and in one of 106 patients (0.9%) who were receiving 2 g/d of imipenem (p<0.005).The 2 g daily dose of imipenem was as effective as the 4 g daily dose. Diarrhea was more frequent in patients receiving cefoperazone, whereas nausea occurred more often with imipenem. No antibiotic-related hemorrhage or nephrotoxicity was observed. Superinfections caused by beta-lactam-resistant, gram-negative bacilli were uncommon, but occurred more frequently with double beta-lactam therapy than with imipenem monotherapy (11 of 268 patients, compared with one of 135 patients; p=0.06). Xanthomonas maltophilia superinfections occurred only in patients receiving imipenem (three of 135 patients, compared with 0 of 268 patients; p=0.03). Imipenem monotherapy was the least expensive therapy.

Conclusion

Cefoperazone and ceftazidime were equally effective when used in combination antibiotic therapy with piperacillin. Twice-daily cefoperazone is less expensive than ceftazidime given three times daily. Monotherapy with imipenem, at a daily dose of 2 g, is as efficacious as double beta-lactam therapy and costs less than combination therapy.

3. Infections in Special Hosts

b. Infections in Organ Transplant Recipients

Randomized, Controlled Trial of Selective Bowel Decontamination for Prevention of Infections Following Liver Transplantation

Title	Randomized controlled trial of selective bowel decontamination for prevention of infections following liver transplantation.
Authors	Arnow PM, Carandang GC, Zabner R, et al.
Reference	Clin Infect Dis 1996;22(6):997–1003.
Disease/Pathogen	Bacterial infections.
Purpose	To compare the conventional prophylaxis with systemic antibiotics with conventional prophylaxis plus oral nonabsorbable antibiotics for selective bowel decontamination (SBD).
Design	Randomized, prospective study.
Patients	69 patients undergoing liver transplants.
Treatment/prophylaxis regimen	Patients were randomly assigned to receive conventional prophylaxis with systemic antibiotics (control patients) or conventional prophylaxis plus oral nonabsorbable antibiotics for SBD (SBD patients).

(continued)

Results   Overall rates of bacterial and/or yeast infections were
                 nearly equal among control patients (42%) and SBD
                 patients (39%). However, the infection rate at SBD key
                 sites (abdomen, bloodstream, surgical wound, and lungs)
                 was lower among patients who received the SBD regimen
                 ≥3 days before transplantation (23%) than among control
                 patients (36%). Administration of the SBD regimen was
                 complicated by gastrointestinal intolerance and noncom-
                 pliance, but not by increased stool colonization with
                 antibiotic-resistant gram-negative bacilli.

Conclusion   Practical problems associated with administering a SBD
                 regimen to patients awaiting cadaver liver transplants
                 limit the regimen's usefulness, but we found a trend
                 toward reduced key site infection when the regimen was
                 given ≥3 days before transplantation.

3. Infections in Special Hosts

c. Infections in Patients with Diabetes

Use of Ampicillin/Sulbactam Vs Imipenem/Cilastatin in the Treatment of Limb-Threatening Foot Infections in Diabetic Patients

Title	Use of ampicillin/sulbactam vs imipenem/cilastatin in the treatment of limb-threatening foot infections in diabetic patients.
Authors	Grayson ML, Gibbons GW, Habershaw GM, et al.
Reference	Clin Infect Dis 1994;18(5):683–693.
Disease/ Pathogen	Foot infections in diabetic patients.
Purpose	To compare the efficacy of imipenem/cilastatin (I/C) and ampicillin/sulbactam (A/S) for initial empirical and definitive parenteral treatment of limb-threatening pedal infection in diabetic patients.
Design	Randomized, double blind trial.
Patients	Patients in the two treatment groups were similar in regard to the severity of diabetes; presence of neuropathy and peripheral vascular disease; site and severity of infection; pathogen isolated; and frequency of osteomyelitis (associated with 68% of the 48 A/S-treated infections, and 56% of the 48 I/C-treated infections).
Follow-up	The major end points of treatment were cure (resolution of soft-tissue infection), failure (inadequate improvement, necessitating a change in antibiotic therapy), and eradication (clearance of all pathogens from the wound and any bone cultures).
Treatment/ prophylaxis regimen	Patients received either I/C (500 mg every 6 hours) or A/S (3 g every 6 hours).

Use of Ampicillin/Sulbactam Vs Imipenem/Cilastatin in the Treatment of Limb-Threatening Foot Infections in Diabetic Patients

(continued)

Results

After 5 days of empirical treatment, improvement was noted in 94% of the A/S and 98% of the I/C recipients. At the end of definitive treatment (days' duration [mean±SD]: 13±6.5 [A/S], 14.8±8.6 [I/C]), outcomes were similar: Cure 81% (A/S) vs 85% (I/C); failure 17% (A/S) vs 13% (I/C); and eradication 67% (A/S) vs 75% (I/C). Treatment failures were associated with the presence of antibiotic-resistant pathogens and possible nosocomial acquisition of infections. The number of adverse events among patients in the two treatment groups was similar: seven in the A/S group (four had diarrhea and three had rash) and nine in the I/C group (five had diarrhea, two had severe nausea, one had rash, and one had seizure).

Conclusion

Efficacy of A/S and I/C is similar for initial empirical, and definitive treatment of limb-threatening pedal infection in patients with diabetes.

Cost-Effectiveness of Ampicillin/Sulbactam Vs Imipenem/Cilastatin in the Treatment of Limb-Threatening Foot Infections in Diabetic Patients

Title	Cost-effectiveness of ampicillin/sulbactam vs imipenem/cilastatin in the treatment of limb-threatening foot infections in diabetic patients.
Authors	McKinnon PS, Paladino JA, Grayson ML, et al.
Reference	Clin Infect Dis 1997;24(1):57–63.
Disease/ Pathogen	Foot infections.
Purpose	To examine the cost effectiveness of ampicillin/sulbactam (A/S) vs imipenem/cilastatin (I/C) in the treatment of limb-threatening foot infections in diabetic patients.
Design	A cost-effectiveness analysis was performed following a double blind, randomized study of ampicillin/sulbactam vs imipenem/cilastatin for the treatment of limb-threatening foot infections in diabetic patients.
Patients	90 diabetic patients with foot infections.
Results	There were no significant differences between the treatments in terms of clinical success rate, adverse-event frequency, duration of study antibiotic treatment, or length of hospitalization. Costs of the study antibiotics, treatment of failures and adverse events, and hospitalization were calculated. Mean per-patient treatment cost in the A/S group was $14,084, compared with $17,008 in the I/C group (p=0.05), primarily because of lower drug and hospitalization costs, and less-severe adverse events in the A/S group. Sensitivity analyses varying drug prices or hospital costs demonstrated that A/S was consistently more cost-effective than I/C.

Cost-Effectiveness of Ampicillin/Sulbactam Vs Imipenem/Cilastatin in the Treatment of Limb-Threatening Foot Infections in Diabetic Patients

(continued)

Conclusion Varying the clinical success rate for each drug revealed that I/C would have to be 30% more effective than A/S to change the economic decisions.

Antibiotic Therapy for Diabetic Foot Infections: Comparison of Two Parenteral-to-Oral Regimens.

Title	Antibiotic therapy for diabetic foot infections: Comparison of two parenteral-to-oral regimens.
Authors	Lipsky BA, Baker PD, Landon GC, et al.
Reference	Clin Infect Dis 1997;24(4):643–648.
Disease/ Pathogen	Foot infections.
Purpose	To compare the efficacy of two antibiotic regimens for treatment of foot infections in diabetic adults.
Design	Prospective, randomized, multicenter trial. Patients with infections requiring hospitalization.
Patients	108 patients with foot infections requiring hospitalization. Patients with osteomyelitis were eligible for the study if the infected bone was to be removed.
Follow-up	For the ofloxacin and aminopenicillin regimens, the mean duration of intravenous therapy was 7.8 and 7.1 days, respectively. The mean duration of oral therapy was 13.2 and 12 days, respectively.
Treatment/ prophylaxis regimen	Patients were randomized to receive either intravenous ofloxacin followed by oral ofloxacin or intravenous ampicillin/sulbactam followed by oral amoxicillin/clavulanate (the aminopenicillin regimen) for 14–28 days.

Results | Of 108 patients enrolled in the study, 88 who were evaluable had various skin and soft-tissue infections, and 24% had osteomyelitis. For the ofloxacin and aminopenicillin regimens, the rate of eradication of pathogens was 78% and 88%, respectively, and the overall rate of clinical cure or improvement was 85% and 83%, respectively.

Conclusion | 3 weeks of therapy with either regimen was well tolerated and effective in treating these diabetic foot infections.

3. Infections in Special Hosts
d. Infections in the Elderly

Meropenem Vs Cefuroxime Plus Gentamicin for Treatment of Serious Infections in Elderly Patients

Title	Meropenem vs cefuroxime plus gentamicin for treatment of serious infections in elderly patients.
Authors	Jaspers CA, Kieft H, Speelberg B, et al.
Reference	Antimicrob Agents Chemother 1998;42(5):1233–1238.
Disease/ Pathogen	Serious infections.
Purpose	To compare the efficacy of and tolerability of meropenem with the combination of cefuroxime-gentamicin (±metronidazole) for the treatment of serious bacterial infections in patients ≥65 years of age.
Design	Randomized, controlled trial, multicenter.
Patients	79 patients 65 years of age or older with serious infections.
Follow-up	70 patients were evaluable for clinical efficacy; the primary diagnoses were as follows: Pneumonia in 41 patients (20 treated with meropenem, 21 treated with cefuroxime-gentamicin); intra-abdominal infection in 10 patients (seven meropenem, three cefuroxime-gentamicin-metronidazole); urinary tract infection (UTI) in 11 patients (six meropenem, five cefuroxime-gentamicin); sepsis syndrome in 7 patients (four meropenem, three cefuroxime-gentamicin); and "other" in one patient (cefuroxime-gentamicin).

Treatment/ prophylaxis regimen	39 patients received meropenem (1 g/8 h), and 40 received cefuroxime (1.5 g/8 h) plus gentamicin (4 mg/kg of body weight daily) for 5–10 days. Metronidazole (500 mg/6 h) could be added to the cefuroxime-gentamicin regimen for the treatment of intra-abdominal infections (n=10).
Results	The pathogens isolated from 18 patients with bacteremia were as follows: Staphylococcus species (n=2), Streptococcus species (n=2), members of the family enterobacteriaceae (n=11), and Bacteroides species (n=3). A satisfactory clinical response at the end of therapy was achieved in 26 of 37 (70%), and 24 of 33 (73%) evaluable patients treated with meropenem and combination therapy, respectively. Clinical success was achieved in 23 of 31 (74%), and 21 of 28 (75%) evaluable patients with infections other than UTIs, respectively. A satisfactory microbiological response occurred in 15 of 22 (68%) patients in the meropenem group compared with 12 of 19 (63%) treated with combination therapy. Renal failure occurred during therapy in two of 39 (5%) meropenem recipients compared with five of 40 (13%) of those treated with combination therapy.
Conclusion	The findings in this small study indicate that meropenem is as efficacious for, and is as well tolerated by elderly patients as the combination of cefuroxime-gentamicin (±metronidazole).

3. Infections in Special Hosts

e. Neonatal Infections

Antibiotic Therapy for Reduction of Infant Morbidity After Preterm Premature Rupture of the Membranes: A Randomized, Controlled Trial.

Title	Antibiotic therapy for reduction of infant morbidity after preterm premature rupture of the membranes: A randomized, controlled trial.
Authors	Mercer BM, Miodovnik M, Thurnau GR, et al.
Reference	JAMA 1997;278:989–995.
Disease/ Pathogen	Intrauterine infection.
Purpose	To determine if antibiotic treatment during expectant management of preterm premature rupture of the membranes (PPROM) will reduce infant morbidity.
Design	Randomized, double blind, multicenter, placebo controlled trial.
Patients	A total of 614 of 804 eligible gravidas with PPROM between 24 weeks' and 0 days' gestation and 32 weeks' and 0 days' gestation, who were considered candidates for pregnancy prolongation, and had not received corticosteroids for fetal maturation or antibiotic treatment within 1 week of randomization.
Follow-up	The composite primary outcome included pregnancies complicated by at least one of the following: Fetal or infant death, respiratory distress, severe intraventricular hemorrhage, stage 2 or 3 necrotizing enterocolitis, or sepsis within 72 hours of birth. These perinatal morbidities were also evaluated individually, and pregnancy prolongation was assessed.

Antibiotic Therapy for Reduction of Infant Morbidity
After Preterm Premature Rupture of the Membranes:
A Randomized, Controlled Trial.

(continued)

Treatment/ prophylaxis regimen	Intravenous ampicillin (2 g dose every 6 hours) and erythromycin (250 mg dose every 6 hours) for 48 hours followed by oral amoxicillin (250 mg dose every 8 hours) and erythromycin base (333 mg dose every 8 hours) for 5 days vs a matching placebo regimen. Group B streptococcus (GBS) carriers were identified and treated. Tocolysis and corticosteroids were prohibited after randomization.
Results	In the total study population, the primary outcome (44.1% vs 52.9%; p=0.04), respiratory distress (40.5% vs 48.7%; p=0.04), and necrotizing enterocolitis (2.3% vs 5.8%; p=0.03) were less frequent with antibiotics. In the GBS-negative cohort, the antibiotic group had less frequent primary outcome (44.5% vs 54.5%; p=0.03), respiratory distress (40.8% vs 50.6%; p=0.03), overall sepsis (8.4% vs 15.6%; p=0.01), pneumonia (2.9% vs 7.0%; p=0.04), and other morbidities. Among GBS-negative women, significant pregnancy prolongation was seen with antibiotics (p<0.001).
Conclusion	The authors recommend that women with expectantly managed PPROM remote from term receive antibiotics to reduce infant morbidity.

Intrapartum Prophylaxis with Ceftriaxone Decreases Rates of Bacterial Colonization and Early-Onset Infection in Newborns

Title	Intrapartum prophylaxis with ceftriaxone decreases rates of bacterial colonization and early-onset infection in newborns.
Authors	Saez-Llorens X, Ah-Chu MS, Castano E, et al.
Reference	Clin Infect Dis 1995;21(4):876–880.
Disease/ Pathogen	Neonatal gram-negative sepsis.
Purpose	To compare the effect of ceftriaxone with no antibiotic prophylaxis (n=394) on oral, rectal, and umbilical colonization and fatality rates among newborn infants.
Design	Prospective study.
Patients	784 high-risk pregnant women
Treatment/ prophylaxis regimen	Patients received a single 1 g dose of ceftriaxone (n=390) or no antibiotic prophylaxis (n=394).

Intrapartum Prophylaxis with Ceftriaxone Decreases Rates of Bacterial Colonization and Early-Onset Infection in Newborns

(continued)

Results	The mean ceftriaxone concentration in umbilical cord blood samples was 26 microgram/mL (range, 9-40 microgram/mL). Compared with infants of untreated mothers, children born to women who were given ceftriaxone were colonized at a lesser rate by gram-negative bacilli (54% vs 35%; p<0.001) and by group B streptococci (54% vs 21%; p=0.03) and endured significantly fewer sepsis-like illnesses in the first 5 days of life (8.1% vs 3.1%; p=0.004). There was also a tendency for them to have fewer episodes of culture-proven early-onset sepsis (2.8% vs 0.5%; p=0.06). Sepsis-related case-fatality rates (0.8% and 0.3%, respectively) were not significantly different.
Conclusion	Although intrapartum administration of a single dose of ceftriaxone to high-risk mothers could be a safe and potentially useful strategy for reducing early-onset neonatal infections, additional information is required before this approach can be recommended for routine prophylaxis.

3. Infections in Special Hosts
f. Neutropenic Fever

Monotherapy with Meropenem Vs Combination Therapy with Ceftazidime Plus Amikacin as Empiric Therapy for Fever in Granulocytopenic Patients with Cancer

Title	Monotherapy with meropenem vs combination therapy with ceftazidime plus amikacin as empiric therapy for fever in granulocytopenic patients with cancer.
Authors	Cometta A, Calandra T, Gaya H, et al.
Reference	Antimicrob Agents Chemother 1996;40(5):1108–1115.
Disease/ Pathogen	Fever in granulocytopenic cancer patients.
Purpose	To compare the efficacy, safety, and tolerance of meropenem monotherapy with those of the combination of ceftazidime plus amikacin for the empirical treatment of fever in granulocytopenic cancer patients.
Design	Prospective, randomized, multicenter study.
Patients	Of 1034 randomized patients, 958 were assessable in the intent-to-treat analysis for response to antibacterial therapy.
Follow-up	The median durations of neutropenia were 16 and 17 days, respectively.
Treatment/ prophylaxis regimen	483 patients received meropenem, and 475 received ceftazidime plus amikacin.

(continued)

Results   A successful outcome was reported in 270 of 483 (56%) patients treated with monotherapy, compared with 245 of 475 (52%) patients treated with the combination group (p=0.2). The success rates in the monotherapy group and the combination group were similar by type of infection (single gram negative bacteremia, single gram positive bacteremia, clinically documented infection, and possible infection). The occurrence of further infections assessed in patients for whom the allocated regimen was not modified did not differ between the two groups (12% in both groups). Mortality due to the presenting infection or further infection was relatively low (eight patients treated with the monotherapy, compared with 13 patients treated with the combination). A total of 1027 patients were evaluable for adverse events; the proportion of those who developed adverse effects was similar between the two groups (29% in both groups), and only 19 (4%) patients in the monotherapy group and 31 (6%) in the combination group experienced an adverse event related or probably related to the study drug. Allergic reactions were the only reason for stopping the protocol antibiotic(s) (three and five patients, respectively).

Conclusion   This study confirms that monotherapy with meropenem is as effective as the combination of ceftazidime plus amikacin for the empiric treatment of fever in persistently granulocytopenic cancer patients, and both regimens were well tolerated.

Discontinuation of Intravenous Antibiotic Therapy During Persistent Neutropenia in Patients Receiving Prophylaxis with Oral Ciprofloxacin

Title	Discontinuation of intravenous antibiotic therapy during persistent neutropenia in patients receiving prophylaxis with oral ciprofloxacin.
Authors	Cornelissen JJ, Rozenberg-Arska M, Dekker AW.
Reference	Clin Infect Dis 1995;21(5):1300–1302.
Disease/ Pathogen	Gram-negative bacterial infection.
Purpose	To evaluate the mortality and morbidity associated with early discontinuation of intravenously administered antibiotics.
Design	Prospective study.
Patients	Patients with persistent neutropenia who responded to a short course of intravenous antibiotic therapy.
Treatment/ prophylaxis regimen	Oral ciprofloxacin as prophylaxis for infection by gram-negative bacteria during the entire neutropenic episode.
Results	The rate of response to either initial or modified intravenous antibiotic therapy was 96% (149 of 156 episodes of fever). 85 patients had an episode of persistent neutropenia (median duration, 7 days; range, 1-36 days) after they responded to treatment. Seven of these patients had recurrent fever, including 2 with bacteriologically documented infections, 4 with probable fungal pneumonia, and 1 with documented pneumonia due to Aspergillus fumigatus. Two patients with probable fungal pneumonia died, while the other infectious episodes resolved completely.

Discontinuation of Intravenous Antibiotic Therapy During Persistent Neutropenia in Patients Receiving Prophylaxis with Oral Ciprofloxacin

(continued)

Conclusion

These results do not support the continuation of intravenous antibiotic therapy for febrile patients with persistent neutropenia who have responded to the antibiotic regimen while receiving prophylaxis with oral ciprofloxacin.

Cefepime/Amikacin Vs Ceftazidime/Amikacin as Empirical Therapy for Febrile Episodes in Neutropenic Patients: A Comparative Study.

Title	Cefepime/amikacin vs ceftazidime/amikacin as empirical therapy for febrile episodes in neutropenic patients: A comparative study.
Authors	Cordonnier C, Herbrecht R, Pico JL, et al.
Reference	Clin Infect Dis 1997;24(1):41-51.
Disease/ Pathogen	Febrile episodes in neutropenic patients.
Purpose	To compare the efficacy and safety of two antibiotic regimens (cefepime plus amikacin or ceftazidime plus amikacin) as first-line therapy for fever in patients with hematologic malignancies and neutropenia.
Design	Randomized, multicenter study.
Patients	A total of 353 patients were randomized according to a 2:1 (cefepime:ceftazidime) ratio. 212 patients in the cefepime group, and 107 in the ceftazidime group (90% of all patients) were evaluable for efficacy.
Follow-up	The mean duration of neutropenia was 26 days.
Treatment/ prophylaxis regimen	Patients received either cefepime [2 g b.i.d.] plus amikacin or ceftazidime 2 g t.i.d. plus amikacin.

Cefepime/Amikacin Vs Ceftazidime/Amikacin as Empirical Therapy for Febrile Episodes in Neutropenic Patients: A Comparative Study.

(continued)

Results
The polymorphonuclear neutrophil count was <100/mm^3 on enrollment for 70% of the patients. The efficacy in both study arms was comparable, although a trend in favor of cefepime was seen in terms of therapeutic success (response rate 27% vs 21% for the ceftazidime group). The overall response rate after glycopeptides were added to the regimens was 60% for the cefepime group, and 51% for the ceftazidime group; the bacterial eradication rates were 81% vs 76%, respectively, and the rates of new bacterial infections were 14% vs 18%, respectively.

Conclusion
The authors conclude that the combination cefepime/amikacin is at least as effective as the reference regimen of ceftazidime/amikacin in this setting.

Sulbactam/Cefoperazone Vs Cefotaxime for the Treatment of Moderate-to-Severe Bacterial Infections: Results of a Randomized, Controlled, Clinical Trial.

Title	Sulbactam/cefoperazone vs cefotaxime for the treatment of moderate-to-severe bacterial infections: Results of a randomized, controlled, clinical trial.
Authors	Li JT, Lu Y, Hou J, et al.
Reference	Clin Infect Dis 1997;24(3):498–505.
Disease/ Pathogen	Moderate-to-severe infections.
Purpose	To compare sulbactam/cefoperazone with cefotaxime in terms of efficacy and safety for the treatment of hospitalized patients with moderate-to-severe bacterial infections.
Design	Randomized, open label, controlled, multicenter study
Patients	207 (88.1%) of the 235 patients enrolled completed the study, and were included in the efficacy and safety evaluations. More than two thirds of the pathogens recovered from these patients produced beta-lactamase.
Treatment/ prophylaxis regimen	103 patients received sulbactam/cefoperazone (2–4 g/d) administered in evenly divided doses every 12 hours by a 30-minute intravenous drip; 104 patients received cefotaxime (6–12 g/d) administered in evenly divided doses every 6 or 8 hours by a 30-minute intravenous drip.

Sulbactam/Cefoperazone Vs Cefotaxime for the Treatment of Moderate-to-Severe Bacterial Infections: Results of a Randomized, Controlled, Clinical Trial.

(continued)

Results   The overall efficacy rates (i.e., cure or markedly improved) were 95% for the sulbactam/cefoperazone group, and 90% for the cefotaxime group, (p=0.186), whereas the bacterial eradication rates were 85% for the sulbactam/cefoperazone group, and 81% for the cefotaxime group (p=0.467). Both drug regimens were well tolerated.

Conclusion   Sulbactam/cefoperazone is effective and safe for the treatment of moderate-to-severe bacterial infections caused mainly by beta-lactamase-producing organisms.

Discontinuation of Antimicrobial Therapy for Febrile, Neutropenic Children with Cancer: A Prospective Study.

Title	Discontinuation of antimicrobial therapy for febrile, neutropenic children with cancer: A prospective study.
Authors	Santolaya ME, Villarroel M, Avendano LF, et al.
Reference	Clin Infect Dis. 1997;25(1):92–97.
Disease/ Pathogen	Fever.
Purpose	To determine the safety of stopping antibiotic therapy on day 3 of therapy in neutropenic children with cancer.
Design	Prospective study.
Patients	Neutropenic children with cancer.
Treatment/ prophylaxis regimen	Children who met predefined criteria for nonbacterial fever were randomized on day 3 to stop (group A) or continue (group B) antibiotic therapy.
Results	A total of 220 children with cancer had 238 episodes of fever and neutropenia; 68 children with 75 episodes met entry criteria for nonbacterial fever (group A, 36; group B, 39). Both groups were comparable in terms of age, gender, oncological disease, chemotherapy status, and initial neutrophil count. Resolution of symptoms occurred in 34 of 36 episodes in group A, and 36 of 39 episodes in group B (p>0.05). No deaths occurred, and bacterial superinfections were uncommon.

Conclusion For children with cancer, as well as episodes of fever and neutropenia without an identifiable bacterial etiology at admission, stopping antibiotic therapy on day 3 was safe and not associated with a higher risk of bacterial super-infections.

Randomized Placebo Controlled Trial of Fluconazole Prophylaxis for Neutropenic Cancer Patients: Benefit Based on Purpose and Intensity of Cytotoxic Therapy.

Title	Randomized placebo controlled trial of fluconazole prophylaxis for neutropenic cancer patients: Benefit based on purpose and intensity of cytotoxic therapy.
Authors	Rotstein C, Bow EJ, Laverdiere M, et al.
Reference	Clin Infect Dis 1999;28(2):331–340.
Disease/ Pathogen	Fungal infections.
Purpose	To compare oral fluconazole (400 mg daily) with placebo as prophylaxis for adult immunosuppressed patients.
Design	Randomized, double blind trial, multicenter.
Patients	Individuals receiving intensive cytotoxic therapy for acute leukemia or autologous bone marrow transplantation.
Treatment/ prophylaxis regimen	Oral fluconazole (400 mg daily) or placebo.

Randomized Placebo Controlled Trial of Fluconazole Prophylaxis for Neutropenic Cancer Patients: Benefit Based on Purpose and Intensity of Cytotoxic Therapy.

(continued)

Results | Although fluconazole prophylaxis did not obviate the need for parenteral antifungal therapy compared with placebo (81 [57%] of 141 vs 67 [50%] of 133, respectively), its use resulted in fewer superficial fungal infections (10 [7%] of 141 vs 23 [18%] of 131, respectively; p=0.02) and fewer definite and probable invasive fungal infections (nine vs 32, respectively; p=0.0001). Fluconazole recipients had fewer deaths attributable to definite invasive fungal infection (one of 15 vs six of 15, respectively; p=0.04) and achieved more frequent success without fungal colonization (52 [37%] of 141 vs 27 [20%] of 133, respectively; p=0.004; relative risk reduction 85%) than did placebo recipients. Patients benefiting the most from fluconazole prophylaxis included those with acute myeloid leukemia who were undergoing induction therapy with cytarabine plus anthracycline-based regimens, and those receiving marrow autografts not supported with hematopoietic growth factors.

Conclusion | Fluconazole prophylaxis reduces the incidence of superficial fungal infection, invasive fungal infection, and fungal infection-related mortality among patients who are receiving intensive cytotoxic chemotherapy for remission induction.

Itraconazole Oral Solution as Prophylaxis for Fungal Infections in Neutropenic Patients with Hematologic Malignancies: A Randomized, Placebo Controlled, Double Blind, Multicenter Trial.

Title	Itraconazole oral solution as prophylaxis for fungal infections in neutropenic patients with hematologic malignancies: A randomized, placebo controlled, double blind, multicenter trial.
Authors	Menichetti F, Del Favero A, Martino P, et al.
Reference	Clin Infect Dis 1999;28(2):250–255.
Disease/ Pathogen	Fungal infections.
Purpose	To evaluate the efficacy and safety of itraconazole oral solution for preventing fungal infections.
Design	Randomized, placebo controlled, double blind, multicenter trial.
Patients	405 neutropenic patients with hematologic malignancies
Treatment/ prophylaxis regimen	Patients were randomly assigned to receive either itraconazole, 2.5 mg/kg every 12 hours (201 patients), or placebo (204 patients).

Itraconazole Oral Solution as Prophylaxis for Fungal Infections in Neutropenic Patients with Hematologic Malignancies: A Randomized, Placebo Controlled, Double Blind, Multicenter Trial

(continued)

Results
Proven and suspected deep fungal infection occurred in 24% of itraconazole recipients, and in 33% of placebo recipients, a difference of 9 percentage points (95% confidence interval [CI] 0.6%-22.5%; p=0.035). Fungemia due to candida species was documented in 0.5% of itraconazole recipients, and in 4% of placebo recipients, a difference of 3.5 percentage points (95% CI 0.5%-6%; p=0.01). Deaths due to candidemia occurred in none of the itraconazole recipients compared with four placebo recipients, a difference of 2 percentage points (95% CI, 0.05%-4%; p=0.06). Aspergillus infection was documented in four itraconazole recipients (one death) and one placebo recipient (one death). Side effects causing drug interruption occurred in 18% of itraconazole recipients and 13% of placebo recipients.

Conclusion
Itraconazole oral solution was well tolerated and effectively prevented proven and suspected deep fungal infection as well as systemic infection and death due to candida species.

*Randomized, Double Blind Clinical Trial of Amphotericin B
Colloidal Dispersion Vs Amphotericin B in the Empirical
Treatment of Fever and Neutropenia*

Title	Randomized, double blind clinical trial of amphotericin B colloidal dispersion vs amphotericin B in the empirical treatment of fever and neutropenia.
Author	White MH, Bowden RA, Sandler ES, et al.
Reference	Clin Infect Dis 1998;27(2):296–302.
Disease/ Pathogen	Fever and neutropenia.
Purpose	To compare amphotericin B colloidal dispersion (ABCD) with amphotericin B in the empirical treatment of fever and neutropenia.
Design	Prospective, randomized, double blind study.
Patients	Patients with neutropenia and unresolved fever after ≥3 days of empirical antibiotic therapy were stratified by age and concomitant use of cyclosporine or tacrolimus. Patients were randomized to receive therapy with ABCD (4 mg/[kg.d]) or amphotericin B (0.8 mg/[kg.d]) for ≤14 days. A total of 213 patients were enrolled, of whom 196 were evaluable for efficacy.

Randomized, Double Blind Clinical Trial of Amphotericin B Colloidal Dispersion Vs Amphotericin B in the Empirical Treatment of Fever and Neutropenia

(continued)

Results	50% of ABCD-treated patients and 43.2% of amphotericin B-treated patients had a therapeutic response (p=0.31). Renal dysfunction was less likely to develop and occurred later in ABCD recipients than in amphotericin B recipients (p<0.001 for both parameters). Infusion-related hypoxia and chills were more common in ABCD recipients than in amphotericin B recipients (p=0.013, and p=0.018, respectively).
Conclusion	ABCD appeared comparable in efficacy with amphotericin B, and renal dysfunction associated with ABCD was significantly less than that associated with amphotericin B. However, infusion-related events were more common with ABCD treatment than with amphotericin B treatment.

Randomized Comparison of Sulbactam/Cefoperazone with Imipenem as Empirical Monotherapy for Febrile Granulocytopenic Patients

Title	Randomized comparison of sulbactam/cefoperazone with imipenem as empirical monotherapy for febrile granulocytopenic patients.
Authors	Winston DJ, Bartoni K, Bruckner DA, et al.
Reference	Clin Infect Dis 1998;26(3):576–583.
Disease/ Pathogen	Febrile neutropenia.
Purpose	To compare sulbactam/cefoperazone with imipenem as empirical monotherapy for febrile, granulocytopenic patients.
Design	Prospective, randomized, controlled trial.
Patients	203 patients.
Treatment/ prophylaxis regimen	101 patients received sulbactam/cefoperazone (2 g/4 g every 12 hours) and 102 patients received imipenem (500 mg every 6 hours).

Randomized Comparison of Sulbactam/Cefoperazone with Imipenem as Empirical Monotherapy for Febrile Granulocytopenic Patients

(continued)

Results
Documented infections were present in 40% of patients treated with sulbactam/cefoperazone and in 39% of patients receiving imipenem. The number of pretherapy gram-positive pathogens (52 isolates) was twice the number of pretherapy gram-negative pathogens (26 isolates). The overall favorable clinical response rates for sulbactam/cefoperazone (91 of 103 patients, or 88%) and imipenem (84 of 104 patients, or 81%) were similar. Both drugs were generally well tolerated. However, diarrhea occurred more often in patients treated with sulbactam/cefoperazone (31 of 101 patients, or 31%, vs 15 of 102 patients, or 15%; p=0.007), while seizures developed only in patients receiving imipenem (0 of 101 patients vs 3 of 102 patients, or 3%). Superinfections developed in 16% of patients in both study groups but were infrequently caused by beta-lactam-resistant gram-negative bacilli (two cases with sulbactam/cefoperazone therapy and six cases with imipenem).

Conclusion
These results support the efficacy and safety of either sulbactam/cefoperazone or imipenem as empirical monotherapy for febrile granulocytopenic patients.

4. Use of Antibiotics

Once Vs Thrice Daily Gentamicin in Patients with Serious Infections

Title	Once vs thrice daily gentamicin in patients with serious infections.
Authors	Prins JM, Buller HR, Kuijper EJ, et al.
Reference	Lancet 1993;341:335–339.
Disease/ Pathogen	General infections.
Purpose	To determine the efficacy and toxicity of an aminoglycoside.
Design	Randomized trial.
Patients	123 patients were enrolled. For efficacy analysis, only those patients were considered in whom treatment with the aminoglycoside was not stopped within 72 h (n=67); toxicity was analysed on patients receiving aminoglycosides for more than 48 h and not using other nephrotoxic medication (n=85).
Treatment/ prophylaxis regimen	Gentamicin 4 mg/kg every day (OD) or gentamicin 1.33 mg/kg three times daily (MD) (with dose-reduction in case of renal dysfunction) were given intravenously.
Additional therapy	In almost all patients, intravenous amoxycillin 1 g every 6 h was also started.

Results

Baseline characteristics were comparable in both arms. A good clinical response was observed in 32/35 (91%) of the OD and in 25/32 (78%) in the MD group (difference 13%, 95% confidence interval [CI] -6.4%–26.9%). Two patients in each group died with uncontrolled infection. An insufficient bacteriological response (persistent positive cultures, resistance, or superinfection) was observed in two patients with OD and three patients with MD. In patients treated for more than 48 h duration of therapy and mean doses were 7 days (1590 mg) and 7.4 days (1672 mg) in OD and MD, respectively. Mean first serum trough/peak levels were 0.6/10.2 mg/L and 1.4/5.2 mg/L. Nephrotoxicity (a rise in serum creatinine of 45 mumol/L or more) developed in 2/40 (5%) in OD, and 11/45 (24%) in MD (p=0.016). Risk factors for nephrotoxicity were duration of therapy and baseline creatinine clearance rate. High-tone audiometry was performed when possible; no significant differences were found in hearing loss (3/12 and 3/11) or prodromal signs of ototoxicity (5/12 and 4/11).

Conclusion

A once-daily dosing regimen of gentamicin is at least as effective as and is less nephrotoxic than more frequent dosing.

Title	Nephrotoxicity and ototoxicity of aztreonam vs amino-glycoside therapy in seriously ill non-neutropenic patients.
Authors	Moore RD, Lerner SA, Levine DP.
Reference	J Infect Dis 1992;165(4):683–688.
Disease/Pathogen	Seriously ill, non-neutropenic patients.
Purpose	To compare aztreonam vs aminoglycoside therapy for the empiric treatment of seriously ill, non-neutropenic patients suspected of aerobic gram-negative bacterial infection.
Design	Randomized, double blind, clinical trial.
Patients	184 seriously ill non-neutropenic patients.
Follow-up	Patient was treated for ≥72 h with the study drug.
Treatment/prophylaxis regimen	92 patients received aminoglycoside therapy, and 92 patients received aztreonam.

Results   Nephrotoxicity, defined by ≥50% increase in baseline serum creatinine, occurred in 12 (15%) of 92 patients receiving aminoglycoside therapy, and one (1%) of 92 patients receiving aztreonam (p<0.004). More severe nephrotoxicity, defined by ≥100% increase in baseline serum creatinine, occurred in six (6.5%) of 92 patients receiving aminoglycoside therapy, and in one of 92 receiving aztreonam (p<0.11). Patients with an elevated baseline total bilirubin level were most likely to develop nephrotoxicity. Auditory toxicity occurred in two (7%) of 28 evaluable patients receiving aminoglycoside therapy and in one (3%) of 33 receiving aztreonam (p<0.58). One patient, who received aminoglycoside, developed vestibular toxicity.

Conclusion   In non-neutropenic patients believed to be at increased risk for renal dysfunction, aztreonam is a less toxic alternative to aminoglycoside therapy for treatment of suspected aerobic gram-negative infection.

A Randomized Comparison of the Safety and Efficacy of Once-Daily Gentamicin or Thrice-Daily Gentamicin in Combination with Ticarcillin-Clavulanate

Title	A randomized comparison of the safety and efficacy of once-daily gentamicin or thrice-daily gentamicin in combination with ticarcillin-clavulanate.
Authors	Gilbert DN, Lee BL, Dworkin RJ, et al.
Reference	Am J Med 1998;105:182–191.
Disease/ Pathogen	General infections.
Purpose	The primary purpose of the clinical trial was to assess the safety and efficacy of once-a-day compared with three-times-a-day gentamicin in patients with serious infections who had protocol-determined peak serum aminoglycoside.
Design	Randomized trial.
Patients	A total of 249 hospitalized patients with suspected or proven serious infections.
Treatment/ prophylaxis regimen	Patients were randomized in a 2:2:1 ratio to gentamicin given three times a day with ticarcillin-clavulanate (TC), gentamicin once a day with TC, or TC alone. The gentamicin once-a-day dosage for patients with estimated creatinine clearance values of ≥80 mL/min was 5.1 mg/kg. With lower creatinine clearance estimates, the mg/kg dosage of gentamicin was decreased, and the dosage intervals (once daily or three times a day) were maintained.

A Randomized Comparison of the Safety and Efficacy of Once-Daily Gentamicin or Thrice-Daily Gentamicin in Combination with Ticarcillin-Clavulanate

(continued)

Results
: Of the total 175 evaluable patients, there were no significant differences found between treatment regimens with respect to clinical or microbiologic efficacy. Bedside audiometry proved impractical, due to the frequency of altered mental state in ill patients. Based on the traditional increase in serum creatinine values from baseline values, no differences in renal toxicity between the treatment groups was identified. When changes in renal function were reanalyzed based on maintaining, as opposed to worsening, of renal function, preservation of renal function was better in the gentamicin once-a-day patients as opposed to the gentamicin three-times-a-day patients, $p<0.01$.

Conclusion
: Gentamicin once-a-day plus TC, gentamicin three times a day plus TC, and TC alone had similar effects in seriously ill hospitalized patients. The incidence of nephrotoxicity was similar in the three treatment groups. Using a nonvalidated post-hoc analysis, renal function was better preserved in gentamicin once-a-day + TC and TC-only patients, as opposed to gentamicin three-times-a-day + TC.

Increasing Immunization Rates Among Inner-City, African-American Children: A Randomized Trial of Case Management.

Title	Increasing immunization rates among inner-city, African-American children: A randomized trial of case management.
Authors	Wood D, Halfon N, Donald-Sherbourne C, et al.
Reference	JAMA 1998;279:29–34.
Disease/ Pathogen	Immunizations.
Purpose	To assess the effectiveness of case management in raising immunization levels among infants of inner-city, African-American families.
Design	Randomized, controlled trial, with follow-up through 1 year of life.
Patients	A representative sample of 419 African-American infants and their families.
Follow-up	Percentage of children with up-to-date immunizations at age 1 year, characteristics associated with improved immunization rates, and cost-effectiveness of case management intervention.
Treatment/ prophylaxis regimen	In-depth assessment by case managers before infants were 6 weeks of age, with home visits 2 weeks prior to when immunizations were scheduled and additional follow-up visits as needed.

Increasing Immunization Rates Among Inner-City, African-American Children: A Randomized Trial of Case Management.

(continued)

Results	A total of 365 newborns were followed up to age 1 year. Overall, the immunization completion for the case management group was 13.2 percentage points higher than the control group (63.8% vs 50.6%; p=0.01). In a logistic model, the case management effect was limited to the 25% of the sample who reported three or fewer well-child visits (odds ratio, 3.43; 95% confidence interval [CI] 1.26–9.35); for them, immunization levels increased by 28 percentage points. Although for the case management group, intervention was not cost-effective ($12,022 per additional child immunized), it was better ($4546) for the 25% of the sample identified retrospectively to have inadequate utilization of preventive health visits.
Conclusion	A case management intervention in the first year of life was effective but not cost-effective at raising immunization levels in inner-city, African-American infants. The intervention was demonstrated to be particularly effective for subpopulations that do not access well-child care. However, currently there are no means to identify these groups prospectively. For case management to be a useful tool to raise immunizations levels among high-risk populations, better methods of tracking and targeting, such as immunization registries, need to be developed.

***Antibiotic Prophylaxis for Infectious Complications
After Therapeutic Endoscopic Retrograde
Cholangiopancreatography: A Randomized, Double Blind,
Placebo Controlled Study.***

Title	Antibiotic prophylaxis for infectious complications after therapeutic endoscopic retrograde cholangiopancreatography: A randomized, double blind, placebo controlled study.
Authors	Byl B, Deviere J, Struelens MJ, et al.
Reference	Clin Infect Dis 1995;20(5):1236–1240.
Disease/ Pathogen	Cholangitis.
Purpose	To examine the efficacy of antibiotic prophylaxis for infectious complications after therapeutic endoscopic retrograde cholangiopancreatography (ERCP).
Design	Randomized, double blind, placebo controlled trial.
Patients	68 clinically evaluable patients underwent 81 therapeutic ERCP procedures.
Follow-up	Clinical success was defined as an absence of fever, cholangitis, and clinical signs of sepsis during the 48 hours after the last dose of piperacillin or placebo.

Antibiotic Prophylaxis for Infectious Complications After Therapeutic Endoscopic Retrograde Cholangiopancreatography: A Randomized, Double Blind, Placebo Controlled Study.

(continued)

Treatment/ prophylaxis regimen	The patients were assigned to receive piperacillin (4 g) or placebo three times daily; prophylaxis was started just before initial ERCP, and was continued until biliary drainage was completely unobstructed (by one or more ERCP procedures); the maximal duration of prophylaxis was 7 days.
Results	Clinical success was documented for 32 (94%) of the 34 patients given piperacillin, and for 24 (71%) of the 34 patients given placebo (odds ratio 6.66; p=0.01). Complete biliary drainage influenced clinical outcome favorably (odds ratio 5; p=0.02). All seven instances of bacteriologic failure (bacteremia) involved patients in the placebo group (p<0.01).
Conclusion	The authors conclude that antimicrobial prophylaxis significantly reduces the incidence of septic complications after therapeutic ERCP among patients presenting with cholestasis.

NIAD Mycoses Study Group Multicenter Trial of Oral Itraconazole Therapy for Invasive Aspergillosis

Title	NIAD Mycoses Study Group multicenter trial of oral itraconazole therapy for invasive aspergillosis.
Authors	Denning DW, Lee JY, Hostetler JS, et al.
Reference	Am J Med 1994;97:135–144.
Disease/ Pathogen	Aspergillosis.
Purpose	To evaluate oral itraconzole in the treatment of aspergillosis.
Design	Multicenter, open study.
Patients	Our study population consisted of 76 evaluable patients.
Follow-up	Response was based on clinical and radiologic criteria plus microbiology, histopathology and autopsy data. Responses were categorized as complete, partial, or stable. Failure was categorized as an itraconazole failure or overall failure. Therapy duration varied from 0.3 to 97 weeks (median 46).
Treatment/ prophylaxis regimen	Patients received oral itraconazole (600 mg/d for 4 days followed by 400 mg/d).

Results

At the end of treatment, 30 (39%) patients had a complete or partial response, and three (4%) had a stable response, and in 20 patients (26%), the protocol therapy was discontinued early (at 0.6–54.3 weeks) because of a worsening clinical course or death due to aspergillosis (itraconazole failure). 23 (30%) patients withdrew for other reasons, including possible toxicity (7%) and death, due to another cause but without resolution of aspergillosis (20%). Itraconazole failure rates varied widely according to site of disease and underlying disease group: 14% for pulmonary and tracheobronchial disease, 50% for sinus disease, 63% for central nervous system disease, and 44% for other sites; 7% in solid organ transplant, 29% in allogeneic bone marrow transplant patients, and 14% in those with prolonged granulocytopenia (median 19 days), 44% in acquired immune deficency syndrome (AIDS) patients, and 32% in other host groups. The relapse rates among those who completed therapy and those who discontinued early for possible toxicity were 12% and 40%, respectively; all were still immunosuppressed.

Conclusion

Oral itraconazole is a useful alternative therapy for invasive aspergillosis with response rates apparently comparable to amphotericin B. Relapse in immunocompromised patients may be a problem. Controlled trials are necessary to fully assess the role of itraconazole in the treatment of invasive aspergillosis.

5. Ongoing Trials

a. Community-Acquired Pneumonia

Prospective Study on the Usefulness of Sputum Gram Stain in the Diagnosis and Initial Therapy of Moderate-to-Severe Community-Acquired Pneumonia (CAP)

Title	Prospective study on the usefulness of sputum gram stain in the diagnosis and initial therapy of moderate-to-severe community-acquired pneumonia (CAP).
Authors	Roson B, Carratala J, Verdaguer R, et al.
Reference	38th Annual ICAAC, San Diego, CA, 1998.
Summary	The value of sputum gram stain in the management of pneumonia is controversial. The objective of our study was to assess the usefulness of sputum gram stain to orientate the diagnosis and the initial antibiotic therapy of CAP. We have prospectively studied 533 consecutive adult patients admitted for moderate-to-severe CAP from February 1995 to May 1997. Spontaneous expectorated sputum samples of good quality (GQS) ($\geq$25 polymorphonuclear cells and <10 squamous cells/LPF) were obtained in 210 patients (39.4%). A predominant single morphotype was seen in 175 of 210 GQS (83.3%). Factors associated with GQS by logistic recession analysis were: Bacterial pneumonia (odds ratio[OR]=9.8; confidence interval [CI] 2.8–34.4), Chronic obstructive pulmonary disease (COPD) (OR=2.5; CI 1.2–5.2), and respiratory failure (OR=2.4; CI 1.3–4.2). The 284 cases in which the etiologic diagnosis was established were used as standard for calculations. The most frequent causative organisms were Streptococcus pneumoniae, 135 cases; Legionella pneumophila, 35 cases; Haemophilus influenzae, 30 cases; and atypical agents, 24 cases. Sensitivity, specificity, and positive and negative predictive values of gram stain for pneumococcal pneumonia were 56.3%, 97.3%, 95%, 71.7%; the corresponding values for H. influenzae pneumonia were 80%, 98.8%, 89.9%, 97.7%, respectively. Overall, 155/175 patients with a predominant single morphotype in a GQS were treated initially with a single antimicrobial agent, and no further modifications were done in 142 of them (91.6%). Our study shows that gram stain of a GQS is highly specific for the diagnosis of

Prospective Study on the Usefulness of Sputum Gram Stain in the Diagnosis and Initial Therapy of Moderate-to-Severe Community-Acquired Pneumonia (CAP)

(continued)

pneumococcal and H. influenzae pneumonia, and that it can be useful in guiding initial antibiotic therapy, avoiding broad-spectrum combination therapy in a large proportion of patients with CAP.

Title	Etiology of community-acquired pneumonia in the elderly.
Authors	Birot P, Didier A, Murris-Espin M, et al.
Reference	38th Annual ICAAC, San Diego, CA, 1998.
Background	Nearly all studies of the etiology of community-acquired pneumonia (CAP) in the elderly show that Streptococcus pneumoniae remains the first agent followed by Hemophilus influenzae. The role of other gram-negative bacilli (GNB) is unclear and a microbial cause is found less often than in younger adults.
Methods	We undertook a multicenter study during a 1-year-period (March 1996–March 1997) in a group of elderly patients (age>65 years) treated as inpatients for CAP across seven medical departments in Toulouse (France). The aim of this study was to determine the causative agents of CAP in this selected population.
Results	We included 136 patients (mean age: 79.4±7.97 years ranging from 65–97 years). 32.6% had received antibiotics before admission. An etiologic diagnosis was obtained in 60 cases (44.1%). The most common pathogens were GNB (others than Hemophilus influenzae) (35%), followed by intracellular bacteria (such as Chlamydia pneumoniae, Legionella pneumophila, and Mycoplasma pneumoniae) (15%) then H. influenzae (11.7%). Staphylococcus aureus (10%) and Streptococcus pneumoniae (8.4%) were less frequent. Bronchoaspiration was performed in 47 cases (34.6%) and provided a diagnosis in 25 (53.2%). Blood cultures was performed on 106 cases (77.9%) and positive on 15 (14.2%). Interestingly, 8 of the 15 positive blood culture specimens identified a GNB as a causative agent.

Conclusions
This study shows that GNB is an important cause of CAP in the elderly. In our population of elderly patients, blood culture was useful not only to identify S. pneumoniae but also bacteremia due to GNB. The low incidence of S. pneumoniae may be related to a frequent antibiotherapy before admission.

5. Ongoing Trials

b. Cystitis

Increasing Prevalence of Antimicrobial Resistance among Uropathogens Causing Acute Uncomplicated Cystitis

Title	Increasing prevalence of antimicrobial resistance among uropathogens causing acute uncomplicated cystitis.
Authors	Gupta K, Scholes D, Stamm WE.
Reference	38th Annual ICAAC, San Diego, CA, 1998.
Background	Many HMOs have implemented guidelines for the management of acute uncomplicated cystitis, which recommend empiric therapy in properly selected patients. The success of this strategy depends in part upon the predictability of the agents causing cystitis, and knowledge of their antimicrobial susceptibility patterns. To date, most studies reporting such information have been based on surveys of laboratory isolates, precluding evaluation of important epidemiological and clinical correlates.
Methods	To assess changes in the prevalence of antimicrobial resistance among uropathogens causing acute uncomplicated cystitis in a well-defined population of women, we conducted a cross-sectional survey of antimicrobial susceptibilities of urine isolates collected over a 5-year-period (1992–1996) from women HMO enrollees 18–50 years of age with an outpatient diagnosis of acute cystitis.

Increasing Prevalence of Antimicrobial Resistance among Uropathogens Causing Acute Uncomplicated Cystitis

(continued)

Results	Escherichia coli and Staphylococcus saprophyticus were the most common uropathogens, comprising 90% of the 4342 urine isolates studied. The prevalence of resistance among E. coli and among all isolates combined was (20% for ampicillin (AMP), cephalothin (CEPH), and sulfamethoxazole in each year studied. The prevalence of resistance to trimethoprim (TMP) and TMP/SMX rose from ≥9% in 1992, to ≥18% in 1996, among E. coli; and from ≥8% to ≥16% among all isolates combined. There was a statistically significant increasing linear trend in the prevalence of resistance from 1992–1996 among E. coli, and among all isolates combined, to AMP, CEPH, TMP and TMP/SMX. On the other hand, the prevalence of resistance to nitrofurantoin (NTF), gentamicin (GENT), and ciprofloxacin (CIP) was 0–2% among E. coli, and <10% among all isolates combined, and did not change significantly over the 5-year- period.
Conclusions	These data reaffirm that E. coli and S. saprophyticus are the most common etiologic agents causing acute cystitis in this well-defined HMO population of women. The prevalence of resistance to TMP/SMX, AMP, and CEPH has increased significantly in the last 5 years, while resistance remains consistently low to NTF, GENT and CIP. These in vitro susceptibility patterns should be considered, along with other factors, such as efficacy, cost, and cost-effectiveness in selecting empiric therapy for acute uncomplicated cystitis in women.

5. Ongoing Trials

c. Cytomegalovirus Disease

Use of CMV Antigenemia and Culture for Detecting Cytomegalovirus Disease in Bone Marrow Transplant Patients

Title	Use of CMV antigenemia and culture for detecting cytomegalovirus disease in bone marrow transplant patients.
Authors	Toso JF, Henshaw NG, Mirrett S, et al.
Reference	98th General Meeting of the American Society for Microbiology, Atlanta, GA, 1998.
Summary	Cytomegalovirus (CMV) disease is a significant cause of morbidity and mortality in bone marrow transplant patients. CMV antigenemia assays (pp65) are now available and have been successfully used as a marker of impending CMV disease, and as a basis for pre-emptive therapy in this setting. We assessed the use of the CMV-vue® (INSTAR Corp.; Stillwater, MN) pp65 antigenemia assay and viral cultures (shell vial and conventional culture) during and 18-month period in the bone marrow transplant unit. A total of 1539 tests were performed on 54 patients. Of the CMV pp65 assays, 4.7% (16 of 341) were positive, whereas 4% (24 of 597) of the CMV shell vial cultures and 1% (6 of 601) of the conventional CMV cultures were positive. When we correlated positive CMV pp65 assays with cultures done within a 30-day period, 60% (6 of 10) of the patients with a positive CMV pp65 assay had a positive CMV culture. From these 6 pp65 positive patients, eight specimens (two bloods, four urines, and two bronchoalveolar lavages) grew CMV within 3 days of a positive CMV pp65 assay. Antiviral therapy was initiated in all of the patients following a positive CMV pp65 assay, with all subsequent CMV cultures remaining negative. These data show that CMV culture is less sensitive than the CMV pp65 assay, and that culture yields no diagnostic information following implementation of antiviral therapy. Because of its lack of clinical utility, the routine use of CMV culture as a predictor of CMV disease in bone marrow transplant patients is not warranted.

5. Ongoing Trials
d. Entercoccal Endocarditis

Entercoccal Endocarditis (EE):
A Co-Operative Study of 178 Cases.

Title	Entercoccal endocarditis (EE): A co-operative study of 178 cases.
Authors	Almirante B, Peña C, Miro JM, et al
Reference	38th Annual ICAAC, San Diego, CA, 1998.
Summary	In order to know the current clinical characteristics, therapy and prognosis, we have reviewed 178 cases of EE (6.6%) among 2680 episodes of infective endocarditis (IE) diagnosed in eight tertiary teaching hospitals in IE diagnosed in eight in Spain between 1975 and 1997. Prevalence of EE increases from 4.8% in the period before 1986 to 7.2% after this year. 123 patients were male (69%), 55 were female (31%). Mean age was 57 years. Infection was nosocomial-acquired in 37 cases (21%). IE affected native valves in 128 cases (72%), prosthetic valves in 36 cases (20%), and was diagnosed in intravenous drug addicts in 14 cases (8%). A previously known underlying cardiopathy was found in 111 cases (62%), and 109 patients (61%) had a chronic underlying condition. A source of infection was suspected in 62 cases (35%), being the most frequent the urinary tract (27 cases). Mean time of clinical symptoms before diagnosis was 28 days (range 1-240 days). The involved valves were the following: Aortic valve in 78 cases (44%), mitral valve in 60 cases (34%), mitral valve in five cases (3%). The most frequent complications were: Congestive heart failure in 83 patients (47%), and septic emboli in 59 (33%). Enterococcus faecalis was identified in 166 cases (93%), E. faecium in nine (5%), and Enterococcus species in three (3%). High level gentamicin resistance (HLGR) was detected in 20 out of 129 (16%) isolates (six of them were streptomycin-susceptible). Ampicillin, penicillin or vancomycin combined with an

aminoglycoside during 4-6 weeks, was used in 135 patient (76%). Ampicillin alone or a double beta-lactam combination was used in the treatment of IE caused by HLGR strains. Surgical valve replacement was needed in 62 patients (34%). Overall mortality was 24%. Factors influencing prognosis were aortic valve IE and congestive heart failure. In conclusion, EE affects aged patients commonly with underlying diseases. Congestive heart failure and septic emboli are frequent. Surgical therapy is needed in 34% of cases. A high mortality rate was observed. Therapeutical options in EE caused by HLGR strains are discussed.

Shortened Duration of Combined Aminoglycoside Synergistic Therapy in Enterococcal Endocarditis

Title	Shortened duration of combined aminoglycoside synergistic therapy in enterococcal endocarditis.
Author	Olaison L, Hogevik H, Alestic K, et al.
Reference	38th Annual ICAAC, San Diego, CA, 1998.
Background	Treatment regimens for enterococcal endocarditis usually recommends 4-6 weeks penicillin G, ampicillinor vancomycin treatment in combination with an aminoglycoside. In clinical practice, however, a shortened aminoglycoside treatment course has often been given without negative consequences. Is it possible to treat enterocollal endocarditis with a 4-6 week beta-lactam or vancomycin treatment course combined with only 2-3 weeks of aminoglycoside therapy?
Methods	A prospective study on infective endocarditis (IE) in Göteborg, Sweden since 1984 and a nation wide prospective study in Sweden, 1995–97 has identified 59 cases treated as enterococcal endocarditis. The Duke criteria of definite endocarditis was fulfilled in 46 (78%) cases and they were further studied. Clinical outcome and antibiotic treatment regimens given were analyzed.

Results

Mortality during treatment was 15% (7/46) and relapse rate 2% (1/40). Of the seven expired patients, three patients received combined treatment until death, and of the remaining four patients, only one had clinical signs of bacteriological failure. This patient was the only case with a relapse, which occurred 2 days after a 28 day penicillin G-treatment course combined with an aminoglycoside during only 2 days. Cardiac surgery during treatment was given median 29 (85%) cured episodes. These episodes had a total duration of antimicrobial treatment ≤28 days in 3 (8%), 29-35 days in nine (23%), 36-42 days in 16 (41%), and >42 days in 11 (28%) episodes, respectively. Combined aminoglycoside treatment was given ≤days in seven (18%), 8-14 days in 14 (33%), 15-21 days in nine (23%), 22-28 days in two (5%), and >28 days in eight (21%) cured episodes, respectively. Mean duration of symptoms pretreatment in cured episodes was 26 (0-119) days as compared to 10 (1-19) days, in episodes with fatal outcome or relapse.

Conclusions

Duration of combined aminoglycoside therapy can be shortened to 2-3 weeks in uncomplicated enterococcal endocarditis episodes without increased risk of relapses. Prosthetic valve endocarditis and long duration of symptoms (>3 months) might require longer combined synergistic aminoglycoside treatment.

5. Ongoing Trials
e. Enterococci

*Nationwide Multicenter Point-Prevalence Study of
Colonization with Vancomycin-Resistant (VRE) and
Ampicillin-Resistant Enterococci (ARE) among Hospitalized
Patients and Non-Hospitalized Persons in Sweden*

Title	Nationwide multicenter point-prevalence study of colonization with vancomycin-resistant (VRE) and ampicillin-resistant enterococci (ARE) among hospitalized patients and non-hospitalized persons in Sweden.
Authors	Torell E, Olsson-Liljequist B, Hoffman BM, et al.
Reference	38th Annual ICAAC, San Diego, CA, 1998.
Background	Recently, ARE and VRE have emerged as nosocomial pathogens worldwide. In Europe, use of the glycopeptide avoparcin as a growth promoter to livestock has been suggested an important factor associated with VRE colonization outside hospitals. In Sweden, all use of antibiotics as growth promoters to livestock was banned already in 1986. Also the use of glycopeptides in Swedish hospitals had decreased. So far, only a few clinical isolates of VRE have been reported. To investigate colonization rates in hospitalized patients and non-hospitalized persons, two studies were performed.
Methods	Study A: Rectal swabs were taken from all patients hospitalized in two wards in each of 27 hospitals nationwide. Study B: Rectal swabs were taken from persons, not previously hospitalized, on admission to 20 hospitals. Registered data included patients' age, sex, prior hospitalization, travel outside Sweden, and prior antibiotic treatment.

***Nationwide Multicenter Point-Prevalence Study of
Colonization with Vancomycin-Resistant (VRE) and
Ampicillin-Resistant Enterococci (ARE) among Hospitalized
Patients and Non-Hospitalized Persons in Sweden***

(continued)

Results   841 fecal samples were analyzed in the study. Patients were hospitalized in intensive care units (21%), surgical (11%), internal medicine (21%), renal (8%), infectious disease (5%), and geriatric units (34%). ARE were found in the fecal flora of 181 patients (21.5%) and VRE in nine patients (1.1%). Antibiotic treatment within 2 weeks (80% vs 47%), prior cephalosporin (31% vs 17.5%) and quinolone (25% vs 9%) exposure were more common in ARE colonized patients, compared to the non-colonized. All VRE colonized patients were from one university hospital, five at the renal unit, and four at a geriatric unit. All nine VRE isolates were Enterococcus faecium of the vanB genotype. PFGE patterns of six isolates were closely related. Two of the patients had been previously treated with vancomycin, and one of the geriatric patients had regular haemodialysis.

Conclusions   The study suggests low prevalence of VRE colonization in Swedish hospitals, and preliminary data indicate low colonization rates in unhealthy individuals. The absence of VRE of the vanA genotype suggests a different epidemiological situation, compared to other European countries.

5. Ongoing Trials

f. Enterococcus Faecium

Long-Term Colonization with Vancomycin-Resistant Enterococcus Faecium

Title	Long-term colonization with vancomycin-resistant Enterococcus faecium.
Authors	Baden L, Thiemke W, Solnik A, et al
Reference	38th Annual ICAAC, San Diego, CA, 1998.
Background	Vancomycin-resistant enterococci (VRE) have become a serious nosocomial problem. Little is known about the persistence of colonization in the non-oncologic, non-intensive care unit patient. At one VA medical center, with about 600 beds, which approximately 70% are chronic care (nursing home and psychiatric), VRE were first encountered in 1993. Over 4 years, VRE-positive patients underwent multiple surveillance stool cultures for infection control purposes; VRE precautions were discontinued after 3 consecutive negative rectal cultures.
Methods	We studied all patients who had stored VRE isolates ≥1 year apart.

Long-Term Colonization with Vancomycin-Resistant Enterococcus Faecium

(continued)

Results

Of 279 patients who had a positive culture for VRE as of 8/5/97, we found 12 patients who had stored VRE isolates recovered ≥1 year apart. Only two patients had active oncologic issues. From these 12 patients, 42 isolates were studied. All were E. faecium with vancomycin MICs ≥256 µg/ml and teicoplanin MICs ≥16 µg/ml. Pulsed field gel electrophoresis (PFGE) was performed on these isolates. Eight clonal groups were identified; 29 of the 42 strains belonged to one genotypic pattern with 12 sub-groups. In seven of the 12 patients, the paired isolates, separated by ≥1 year, were genotypically indistinguishable or closely related by PFGE patterns. One patient excreted a genotypically indistinguishable clone for 38 months. Three patients had been deemed cleared of VRE (by three consecutive negative rectal cultures) but were later found to be VRE-positive. For two of these three, the recrudescing isolate was genotypically related to their earlier isolate.

Conclusions

Based on the genotypic patterns, VRE most likely persisted at undetectable levels in the gastrointestinal tract in seven of the 12 patients. However, re-infection from environmental sources cannot be excluded. These data suggest that colonization with VRE may persist for years, even if intercurrent surveillance stool cultures are negative for VRE.

5. Ongoing Trials

g. Fungal Burn Wound Infections

Epidemiology and Clinical Characteristics of Fungal Burn Wound Infections

Title	Epidemiology and clinical characteristics of fungal burn wound infections.
Authors	Clancy CJ, Farrell KJ, Nguyen MH.
Reference	38th Annual ICAAC, San Diego, CA, 1998.

| Summary | The introduction of potent topical antibacterial agents in routine burn wound care has reduced morbidity and mortality due to bacterial infections. This has been accompanied by an increase in fungal burn wound infections. We describe six burn patients who developed invasive fungal infections. The median age was 42 years (31–59 years). One patient had chronic obstructive pulmonary disease (COPD), and one patient had diabetes; two patients were alcoholics. All patients were burned by flames (four in house fires, two in campfires). Two patients were rolled in the dirt after their burns. Four patients sustained ≤25% total body surface area (TBSA) burns, and two sustained ≥75% TBSA burns. All were either second or third degree. Topical antibiotic therapy with sulfamylon or silvadene was applied in all patients. Five patients also received broad-spectrum antibiotics. Fungal wound infections were suspected in three patients who had new black eschars (two) or graft failure (one). Histopathology of wounds revealed invasion of subcutaneous tissue by hyphae in five cases. Hyphal invasion of blood vessels or muscle were noted in two patients. The median time from burn to clinical onset of infection was 14 days (5–32) days. Fungi recovered included Fusarium (four) and Candida albicans (one); Geotrichum and Rhizopus were isolated with Fusarium in one case. All patients received amphotericin B (AmB) or liposomal formulations of AmB. two patients underwent amputation, and three patients received extensive debridements of their wounds. One patient did not receive further surgical debridement; she died with Fusarium fungemia and multi-system organ failure 6 days after completing a 2-gram course of AmB. Three of six patients died; two patients became fungemic, and died of disseminated fusariosis. Extent of burn was the |

major prognostic indicator for mortality. All patients with ≥75% TBSA burns died of disseminated fungal infections. All survivors had prolonged hospital stay of ≥2 months for antifungal therapy and repeated debridement. In conclusion, fungi have emerged as major pathogens in burn wound infections in the era of potent topical antibacterial therapy. Invasive infections are associated with significant morbidity and mortality. The key to successful therapy is aggressive debridement in conjunction with prolonged antifungal therapy.

5. Ongoing Trials

h. Haemophilus Influenza

Marked Variability of β-Lactam Resistance in H. Influenzae from Nine Geographically Distinct Countries

Title	Marked variability of β-lactam resistance in H. influenzae from nine geographically distinct countries.
Authors	Davidson RJ, McGeer A, Porter-Pong S, et al.
Reference	38th Annual ICAAC, San Diego, CA, 1998.
Summary	Prior to 1972, Haemophilus influenzae was uniformly susceptible to ampicillin. However, the increasing prevalence of plasmid mediated TEM-1 and ROB-1 β-lactamases, and to a lesser extent, altered penicillin binding proteins have resulted in high rates of penicillin resistance in some countries. Currently, >40% of isolates are penicillin resistant in the United States. We report here on the prevalence of antimicrobial resistance in H. influenzae isolated from nine distinct geographic regions in the world. 565 H. influenzae strains from nine countries: Canada, Germany, Greece, Australia, Korea, Poland, France, Venezuela, and South Africa were collected and submitted to the Mount Sinai Hospital microbiology laboratory for analysis. Isolates were tested for the production of ß-lactamase by the cefinase disk methods. Minimal inhibitory concentrations (MIC) to ampicillin, amoxicillin-clavulanate, cefaclor, cefprozil, loracarbef, cefuroxime, and erythromycin, were determined using a microbroth dilution technique. Overall, approximately 18% of H. influenzae strains produced a β-lactamase. However, <3% of strains from Venezuela, Poland, and Germany were producers. Approximately 30% of strains from Canada produces a β-lactamase, and >40% from France and Korea. Predictably, 18% of strains were resistant to ampicillin with the rates mirroring the prevalence of β-lactamase producing strains in each region. No amoxicillin-clavulanate resistant strains were isolated. 4% of isolates were intermediately resistant to cefaclor and 1.5% were resistant. 4% and 3% of isolates were intermediately resistant to cefprozil and loracarbef, respectively. Approximately 1% of isolates were fully resistant to cefprozil or loracarbef. Only isolate was found to

have intermediate resistance to cefuroxime. Resistant breakpoints have not been determined for erythromycin in H. influenzae. The MIC_{90} to erythromycin was 8 mg/l. The majority of all the currently available antimicrobials used for the treatment of H. influenzae infections continue to have excellent activity. Understanding the reason for the marked variation in β-lactamase production and ampicillin resistance from country to country may help us better understand how to better utilize antimicrobial agents.

5. Ongoing Trials

i. Intra-Abdominal Infections

The Safety and Efficacy of Sequential (IV to PO) Ciprofloxacin (CIP) Plus Metronidazole (MET) Vs Piperacillin/Tazobactam (PIP/TAZO) in the Treatment of Patients with Complicated Intra-Abdominal (INTRAAB) Infections

Title	The safety and efficacy of sequential (IV to PO) ciprofloxacin (CIP) plus metronidazole (MET) vs piperacillin/tazobactam (PIP/TAZO) in the treatment of patients with complicated intra-abdominal (INTRAAB) infections.
Authors	Cohn S, Haverstock D, Kowalsky S, et al
Reference	38th Annual ICAAC, San Diego, CA, 998.
Summary	In a multicenter, randomized, double blind trial, the efficacy of IV CIP (400mg q 12h) + IV MET (500mg q6h) vs IV PIP/TAZO (3.375g q6h) was compared in 459 hospitalized adults with complicated INTRAAB infections. After 48h, IV antibiotics could be switched to oral (PO) therapy, based on improvement and PO tolerability. Upon discharge, all patients could receive PO antibiotics (unblinded phase), at the investigator's discretion, for ≤14 days. Overall clinical response (i.e., worst response of end-of-therapy and 3-5 week post-therapy follow-up) was the primary efficacy measure. A total of 282 patients (151 CIP, 131 PIP/TAZO) were efficacy-valid; PO was given to 96 (64%) ciprofloxacin/metronidazole (CIP/MET) and 75 (57%) PIP/TAZO patients. PO CIP/MET was given most often during the unblinded outpatient phase. Patients were mostly male (63%), Caucasian (61%), and in good/fair health (90%) with a mean age of 48 yrs (range: 1888) and mean Acute Physiology and Chronic Health Evaluation (APACHE) II score of 9.6 (range 0-32). The most common diagnoses were appendicitis (33%), "other" INTRAAB infection (29%), and abscess (25%). Escherichia coli and Bacteroids fragilis were isolated most frequently. Overall, clinical resolution rates were statistically superior for CIP/MET at 74% (99/134) vs 63% (73/116) for PIP/TAZO

The Safety and Efficacy of Sequential (IV to PO) Ciprofloxacin (CIP) Plus Metronidazole (MET) Vs Piperacillin/Tazobactam (PIP/TAZO) in the Treatment of Patients with Complicated Intra-Abdominal (INTRAAB) Infections

(continued)

(C19,=0.03,0.23). Likewise, for CIP/MET patients switched to PO therapy, overall clinical resolution rates were superior to IV/PO switch PIP/TAZO patients: 85% (69/81), and 70% (47/67), respectively. Post-surgical wound infections were also found less often in CIP/MET- (11%) vs PIP/TAZO-treated patients (19%) (p=0.04). Duration of hospitalization was shorter for CIP (14 d) vs PIP/TAZO 917 d) (p=0.16). Drug-related adverse event rates were similar in both groups, CIP/MET was significantly better clinically than PIP/TAZO in the treatment of patients with complicated INTRAAB infections.

5. Ongoing Trials

j. Nosocomial Infections

Nosocomial Infections in Elderly and Very Elderly Patients: A Factor Influencing the Length of Stay and Mortality in a Short-Stay Admission Unit.

Title	Nosocomial infections in elderly and very elderly patients: A factor influencing the length of stay and mortality in a short-stay admission unit.
Authors	De Otero J, Ferrer-Ruscalleda L, Sandiumenge M, et al.
Reference	38th Annual ICAAC, San Diego, CA, 1998.

Summary	Age has been identified as a risk factor for nosocomial infection (NI). Moreover, the role that NI plays, as a major factor, influencing the stay and the mortality in short stay admission units (<7 d admission) for elderly (65–75 year-old [E]) and very elderly (>75 year-old [VE]) population needs to be clearly established. The aim of this study was to analyze the incidence rate of NI in E and VE patients during two consecutive winter periods (1996 and 1997). We also analyzed the contribution of NI to length of stay and mortality. In 1996, 31 E patients were compared with 58 VE patients. Patients with <1 day of hospitalization were excluded. The following data were prospectively collected: Age, sex, length of hospital stay, number and site of NI and hospital deaths. Median age was 72 y (E) and 82.5 y (VE). Length of hospital stay was 7 d and 8 d, respectively (p NS). Incidence of NI was 12.9 and 8.6 per 100 patients (p NS) and 1.53 and 0.82 per 100 days of admission (p NS). Only one patient (E) had more than one episode of NI. Sites of NI were: urinary tract infection (UTI) (50% vs 20%), bacteremia (25% vs 20%), respiratory infection (25% vs 60%); none of these differences reached statistical significance. Mortality rate for infected patients was higher (25% vs 2.5%; p=0.03). Baseline characteristics of patients studied in 1997 (E patients n=26, and VE patients n=62) were similar, except for a longer stay in VE patients (8.5 d vs 7 d; p=0.03). Results in 1997 also showed a longer length of stay and a higher mortality rate in infected patients (15 d vs 7 d, p=0.03; and 28.6 vs 2.5.

Nosocomial Infections in Elderly and Very Elderly Patients: A Factor Influencing the Length of Stay and Mortality in a Short-Stay Admission Unit.

(continued)

p=0.03, respectively). Our results suggest that in a short stay admission unit: 1) the incidence of NI is not different between E and VE patients; 2) NI is associated with a longer hospital stay; 3) NI is associated with a higher mortality.

5. Ongoing Trials

k. Oral or Intravenous Antibiotics

A Double Blind, Randomized Trial of Oral or Intravenous Antibiotics for Empirical Therapy of "Low Risk" Fever and Neutropenia (F=N=) in Cancer Patients

Title	A double blind, randomized trial of oral or intravenous antibiotics for empirical therapy of "low risk" fever and neutropenia (F=N=) in cancer patients.
Authors	Freifeld A, Marchigiani D, Lewis L, et al.
Reference	36th Annual IDSA Meeting, Denver, CO 1998.
Summary	Broad-spectrum oral antibiotics may be an alternative to traditional IV therapy of F+N+ in cancer patients at "low risk" for complications. We conducted a double blind, randomized trial of 280 episodes of "low risk" F+N+ defined by absolute neutrophil count (ANC) expected to return to >500/mm^3 within 10 days, and absence of medical comorbidity (i.e., no hypotension, or abdominal, neurologic, pulmonary changes), in patients who could swallow pills. Of 232 evaluable episodes, 116 were randomized to oral ciprofloxacin (750mg q8h) = amoxicillin/clavulanate (500mg q8h) and 116 to standard IV ceftazidime monotherapy (90 mg/kg/d divided q8h). Oral or IV placebo was given in addition to active drugs. All were hospitalized. Patient age, sex, and underlying disease (70% solid tumors) were comparably distributed in both groups. Mean ANC on entry<100mm^3. Mean duration of N= was 3.5 d in the oral vs 3.8 d in the IV study group. Over 90% were receiving a cytokine at entry. Documented infections occurred in 40% of IV and 31% of oral episodes, with 19 total bloodstream infections. 72% of oral and 67% of IV episodes were successfully managed with initially-assigned antibiotic regimen (p=0.48). Success with modification (addition to or change of antimicrobial regiment to expand coverage) occurred in 15% of oral and <1% of IV episodes (p<0.001), so that changes (modification + failure/intolerance) occurred in 28% of oral and 33% of IV episodes overall (p=0.48, two oral and six IV arm patients

A Double Blind, Randomized Trial of Oral or Intravenous Antibiotics for Empirical Therapy of "Low Risk" Fever and Neutropenia (F=N=) in Cancer Patients

(continued)

required switch to an IV "rescue regimen" to contain infection. No deaths occurred. Inability to tolerate oral medications due to nausea, vomiting, diarrhea of mucositis prevented completion of oral therapy in 8% vs 15% receiving oral placebo vs active oral antibiotics (p=0.07). Empirical oral antibiotic therapy with ciprofloxacin+ amoxicillin/clavulante may be employed safely and effectively in patients hospitalized with "low risk" F+N+, with close follow-up for required modifications or oral intolerance. "Low risk" criteria employed to define this population accurately predicted those who had few complications during F+N+.

5. Ongoing Trials
1. Otitis Media

Oral Ciproflaxacin (CP) Vs Topical Oflaxacin (OFX) for Treatment of Chronic Suppurative Otitis Media (CSOM)

Title	Oral ciproflaxacin (CP) vs topical oflaxacin (OFX) for treatment of chronic suppurative otitis media (CSOM).
Authors	Esposito E, D'Errico G, Noviello S, et al.
Reference	38th Annual ICAAC, San Diego, CA, 1998.

Summary — Oral CP was compared to topical OFX for treatment of CSOM in an open, randomized trial. 140 outpatients over 18 years (age range 18–66) affected by CSOM without cholesteatoma or mastoiditis and with documented bacterial infection caused by micro-organisms "in vitro" sensitive to both CP and OFX were enrolled. Diagnosis was stated according to the following criteria: The otitis media had lasted at least 3 years, purulent otorrhea had recurred at least once annually, and recurrent episodes of purulent otorrhea had been constant for at least 15 days. Exclusion criteria were pregnancy and allergy to quinolones. 71 patients were randomly assigned to receive oral CP (750 mg b.i.d.) and 69 patients were assigned to receive typical OFX (300 mcg/ml solution, 5–6 drops b.i.d., for 7–14 days). Clinical controls by microtoscopy and bacteriological examinations of the ear middle fluid were always performed before, during (every 3 days) and after (24 hours and 14 days) the end of the treatment. Pseudomonas aeruginosa was isolated in 55% of patients; Staphlococcus aureus in 35.7 and other micro-organisms in 9.3%. The following clinical and bacteriological results were obtained:

Antibiotic	No. Pts	Cure/Eradication	Failure/Persistance
CP	71	47 (66.2%)	24 (33.8%)
OFX	69	59 (85.5%)	10 (14.5%)

No side effect was recorded for any patient, and no impairment of the hearing detectable by audiometric tests related to local or oral therapy was observed.Topical OFX is safe and more effective than oral CP (p<0.005) in the treatment of CSOM occurring in adult patients.

5. Ongoing Trials
m. Peritonitis

Multicenter, Randomized, Clinical Trial of Piperacillin Plus Tazobactam (TAZ) and Amikacin (AMK) in the Treatment of Severe Generalized Peritonitis (SGP)

Title	Multicenter, randomized, clinical trial of piperacillin plus tazobactam (TAZ) and amikacin (AMK) in the treatment of severe generalized peritonitis (SGP).
Authors	Dupont H, Carbon C, Carlet J, et al.
Reference	Antimicrob Agents Chemother 2000;44:2028–2033.
Summary	In a randomized trial conducted in 35 centers, we compared the clinical efficacy and saftey of piperacillin plus tazobactam (TAZ) alone (monotherapy [MT]) vs those of TAZ combined with amikacin (AMK) (combined therapy [CT]) for the treatment of severe generalized peritonitis (SGP). Primary analysis consisted of blind assessment by an independent committe of the failure rate 30 days after the end of treatment in the modified intent-to-treat (ITT) analysis (mITT) population. Of the 241 patients with suspected SGP randomized into the study, 227 were eligible for ITT analysis, including 204 (99 in the MT group and 105 in the CT group with confirmed SGP (mITT population). A total of 159 patients were eligible for per-protocol (PP) analysis. The clinical failure rates were equivalent in the mITT and PP populations (MT vs CT): 56% vs 52%, (odds ratio [OR] 0.87; 90% confidence interval [CI]; 0.6–1.27) for mITT and 49% vs 49% (OR 1.03; 90%

Multicenter, Randomized, Clinical Trial of Piperacillin Plus Tazobactam (TAZ) and Amikacin (AMK) in the Treatment of Severe Generalized Peritonitis (SGP)

(continued)

CI; 0.67–1/59) for PPF analysis. Mortality rates (ITT population, 19%; PP population, 21%) and overall adverse event rates (ITT population, 55%; PP population, 54%) were also similar. Six patients (three in MT group and three in the CT group) developed acute renal failure. In conclusion, the addition of AMK to TAZ does not seem to be necessary for the treatment of SGP, even after adjustment for the simplified acute physiology score (SAPS II) and type of SGP.

5. Ongoing Trials

n. Pertussis

Increased Reporting of Pertussis Cases Among Adolescents and Adults in the United States: An Update on the National Pertussis Surveillance Data.

Title	Increased reporting of pertussis cases among adolescents and adults in the United States: An update on the national pertussis surveillance data.
Authors	Guris D, Bardenheier B, Bisgard K, et al.
Reference	38th Annual ICAAC, San Diego, CA, 1998.
Introduction	In recent years, the reported pertussis incidence among adolescents and adults has increased substantially in the U.S. Pertussis epidemics occur every 3-4 years. During the last epidemic year, 1996, the highest number of pertussis cases (7796) since 1967 was reported with an incidence of 2.9 per 100,000 population. Of these cases, 44% occurred among persons aged ≥10 years. To evaluate trends in pertussis in the U.S., we analyzed national pertussis surveillance data from 1995-1997.
Methods	Epidemiologic data on pertussis cases reported to the National Notifiable Diseases Surveillance System and Supplementary Pertussis Surveillance System at the Centers for Disease Control were reviewed.

Increased Reporting of Pertussis Cases Among Adolescents and Adults in the United States: An Update on the National Pertussis Surveillance Data.

(continued)

Results

In 1997, a total of 6315 cases of pertussis were reported (provisional), representing a 19% reduction in the number of cases reported for 1996. However, the number of cases reported in 1997 was 23% higher than in 1995, the previous endemic year. In 1997, 43% of reported cases were aged <5 years, 11% were aged 5–9 years, and 46% were aged ≥10 years. Compared with 1996, in 1997 the smallest reduction (9%) in the number of reported cases was among those aged ≥20 years and the greatest reduction (30%) was among cases aged 1–4 years. States (Idaho, Vermont, New Hampshire, New Mexico, Colorado, Massachusetts, Minnesota, and Washington) with a high reported incidence of pertussis in recent years have continued to report a high incidence of pertussis in 1997 (>7 cases per 100,00). In 1997, 90% of the cases aged ≥10 years had paroxysms, 38% had whoop, 51% had post-tussive vomiting, 2% had pneumonia, and 2% were hospitalized.

Conclusions

Compared to the peak year of 1996, the overall number of pertussis cases decreased in 1997. This decrease was lowest among adolescents and adults, who represent nearly half of all reported cases. However, consistent with the recent upward trend of reported pertussis cases, the number of cases in 1997 was higher than the number of cases in previous endemic year, 1995. Further implementation of the recommended pertussis prevention and control strategies (i.e., timely vaccination of young children, early diagnosis and treatment of cases, and early prophylaxis of contacts) yield only marginal benefits in reducing the occurrence of disease.

5. Ongoing Trials

o. Pneumococcal Resistance

Sequential Surveillance of Antimicrobial Resistance in the United States: Streptococcus Pneumoniae, Haemophilus Influenzae, and Moraxella Catarrhalis (1997–1998 Vs 1996–1997).

Title	Sequential surveillance of microbial resistance in the United States: Streptococcus pneumoniae, Haemophilus influenzae, and Moraxella catarrhalis (1997-1998 vs 1996-1997).
Authors	Thronsberry C, Mickey ML, Diakun DR, et al.
Reference	38th Annual ICAAC, San Diego, CA, 1998.
Summary	Pneumococcal resistance to several antimicrobial agents can develop rapidly. Therefore, the ability to monitor the activity of newly released agents is important. Since the release of levofloxacin (LEVO) in January 1997, we have systematically tracked pneumococcal susceptibility to levofloxacin and seven other antimicrobials against common respiratory pathogens. In 1997-1998, penicillin (PEN) non susceptibility (MIC ≥0.125 µ/ml) in 2240 strains of Streptococcus pneumoniae (SP) was 36% [22% intermediate (I), 14% resistant (R)], compared to 34% nonsusceptible (20% I, 14% R) in 1996-1997. Clarithromycin resistance increased from 18%, to 23% in SP. In 1997–1998 blood isolates, 19% of SP were not susceptible to PEN (19% I, 10% R), compared with 29.8% (24.3% I, 15.5% R) in respiratory isolates. For PEN-resistant SP (MIC ≥2 µg/ml), nonsusceptibility (I+R) for other antimicrobials was 93% for amoxicillin-clavulanate (AC), 80% for ceftriaxone (CTX), 98% for cefuroxime (CUX), 71% for azithromycin (AZ), and clarithromycin (CLAR), and 93% fortrimethroprim-sulfamethoxazole (SXT); all SP were susceptible to vancomycin (VAN) and LEVO. For AC, CUX, VAN, and LEVO, these rates among PEN-resistant isolates were comparable to those in 1996–1997, and there was an increase in CLAR resistance (10%) and CTX resistance (7%). AZ and SXT were not tested in 1996-1997. Resistance in the other respiratory organisms, Haemophilus influenzae (HI)

(continued)

and Moraxella catarhalis (MC), has remained relatively constant between the 1996-1997 and 1997-1998 studies. Both organisms are still 100% susceptible to LEVO, CTX, and CUX, and the percent of orgamisms producing ß-lactamase is comparable to the 1996-1997 study (33.2% vs 33.4% for HI, and 91% for MC). While pneumococcal resistance to many antimicrobials continues to increase, LEVO and VAN have maintained a high level of activity. Ongoing surveillance of pneumococci for resistance to fluoroquinolones, vancomycin, and other agents is imperative.

5. Ongoing Trials

p. Pseudomonas Aeruginosa Bacteremia

Pseudomonas Aeruginosa Bacteremia: A Multicentric Spanish Survey.

Title	Pseudomonas aeruginosa bacteremia: A multicentric Spanish survey.
Authors	Ezpeleta C, Martinez J, Larrea I, et al
Reference	38th Annual ICAAC, San Diego, California, 1998.
Summary	Nosocomial bacteremia is a useful indicator of overall changes in nosocomial infections. The study of bloodstream infections is not subject to some of the difficulties involved in defining infection at other sites. High case-fatality ratios have characterized bacteremia associated with Pseudomonas aeruginosa.
Objective	To assess epidemiological features of P. aeruginosa bacteremia in Spain, and to determine by means of univariate statistical analysis factors influencing prognosis.
Methods	A prospective, multicentric survey of bacteremia (34 hospitals) was carried out between January 94–July 97 by means of 4, EPSIS-DATA (a soft-ware program developed by the Nosocomial Infection Study Group of the Spanish Society of Infectious Diseases and Clinical Microbiology). It has been designed to collect under common criteria bacteremia cases from Spanish hospitals. Overall, 5000 cases of bacteremia have been prospectively followed during this period.
Statistical analysis	Invariant analysis of prognostic factors was performed with EPINFO (CDC) Chi square/OR.

Pseudomonas Aeruginosa Bacteremia:
A Multicentric Spanish Survey.

(continued)

Patients	72.51% males, the most frequent age group >60 y (59.71%). Underlying illnesses: Neoplasia (32.23%), HIV (8%). Predisposing conditions: ICU (23%), surgery (25%), bladder catheterization (36%), antibiotics (43%), intravenous lines (52% fever was present in 89.57% of cases, and rigors in 33.65%). Neutropenia (<1000 PNL) was present in 11% of cases. Sources of bacteremia: Urinary tract (22.75%), respiratory (20.85%), primary (18%), catheter-related (6.16%), surgical site (2.84%). Bacteremias were monomicrobial in 181 cases, and polymicrobial in 30 cases. 3.79% of isolates were recovered after 7 days of incubation. Antibiotic susceptibilities: Amikacin 86%, ceftazidime 86%, fiprofloxacin 83%, imipenem 71%, gentamicin 45%. The antibiotic therapy was appropriate in 93.36% of cases. In 3.55% of cases, the correct antibiotic therapy was started >4 days after blood cultures were obtained. Ceftazidime (67 p), amikacin (956 p) and ciprofloxacin (40 p) were the most frequent antibiotics employed. An association of two antibiotics was used in 70% of cases. Crude mortality until the end of the episode: 26.54%. Mortality was related to age>60 y odds ratio (OR)=2.58; p=0.0076; rapidly fatal underlying illness OR=6.4; p=0.0025; incorrect antibiotic therapy OR=5.06; p=0.0025; and respiratory source of bacteremia OR=2.9; p=0.0027.
Results	In 211 cases (3.96%) P. aeruginosa was recovered from blood. 58.77% cases were hospital-acquired, and 40.28% community-acquired.

5. Ongoing Trials

q. Staphylococcus Aureus

A Randomized, Double Blind, Placebo Controlled Clinical Trial of Intranasal Mupirocin Ointment (IM) for Prevention of S. aureus Surgical Site Infections (SSI)

Title	A randomized, double blind, placebo controlled clinical trial of intranasal mupirocin ointment (IM) for prevention of S. aureus surgical site infections (SSI).
Authors	Perl TM, Cullen JJ, Pfaller MA, et al.
Reference	36th Annual IDSA Meeting, Denver, CO 1998.
Summary	Staphylococcus aureus causes 25% of SSI. These infections increase morbidity, length of stay, and costs. Several studies demonstrated that IM eliminates S. aureus nasal carriage, and prevents infections in specific patient populations. To date, IM's efficacy for preventing S. aureus SSI has not been tested in a placebo controlled, clinical trial. We performed a randomized, double blind, placebo controlled trial to determine whether IM reduces the incidence of S. aureus SSI. 3909 patients who had a cardio-thoracic (18.4%), general (47.6%), vascular (10.2%), neurologic (18.9%), or complicated gynecologic (4.9%) operations at the University of Iowa (91.6%) and the Iowa City VA (8.4%) were enrolled and met inclusion criteria. Enrolled patients had cultures of the anterior nares obtained pre- and post-operatively, and were followed weekly for 4 weeks after the operation. A SSI was defined using modified CDC criteria. The mean age of patients was 54.7 years, 96.5% were Caucasian, 48.4% were females, and 23.2% carried S. aureus in the anterior nares. The S. aureus nasal carriage rates were similar among patients admitted to different services. Overall, 362 rates were similar among patients admitted to different services. Overall, 362 (9.3%) patients acquired SSIs of whom 90 (2.3%) were infected with S. aureus. On average, SSIs developed 18.4 days after the procedure. Among patients with S. aureus SSI, 42/90 (46.7%) carried S. aureus intransally (relative risk [RR]=2.9, p<0.0001). Molecular typing revealed that 86% of patients who carried S. aureus were infected with their own strain. Final study results will be available shortly.

5. Ongoing Trials

r. Staphylococcal Infective Endocarditis

Treatment of Staphylococcal Infective Endocarditis (IE) with Fusidic Acid

Title	Treatment of staphylococcal infective endocarditis (IE) with fusidic acid.
Authors	Leroy O, Millaire A, Klug D, et al.
Reference	38th Annual ICAAC, San Diego, CA, 1998.
Summary	In order to assess the efficacy of fusidic acid for therapy of staphylococcal IE, we retrospectively collected, in a 10-year period (1988–97), all patients exhibiting definite IE, according to Duke criteria and receiving such an antimicrobial agent. 25 patients (18 men and 7 women; mean age=57.8 years) were enrolled. The definite diagnosis of IE was established on the basis of pathological criteria (n=12) and clinical criteria (n=13). In 18 cases, IE was pacemaker-associated. In the remaining cases, IE involved native valve(s) (n=5), ventricular septal defect (n=1) and prosthetic valve (n=1). Causative organisms were S. aureus (n=8), S. epidermidis (n=15), S. capitis (n=1) and Staphylococcus haemolyticus (n=1). In 10 cases, Staphylococcus species was meticillin resistant. 17 patients exhibited IE-associated metastatic infections (n=27) mainly involving lung (n=12) and bone (n=6). In 10 patients, fusidic acid was only used by IV route, in association with glycopeptide (n=7), oxacillin (n=2) or quinolone. The mean duration of this therapy was 13 days. In five cases, fusidic acid, mainly associated with oxacillin, was used by IV route (mean duration=12 days followed by oral route (mean duration=20 days). In the remaining 11 cases, fusidic acid was only administered by oral route as a relay or intravenous therapy, based on other antimicrobial agents. In such cases, fusidic acid was mainly associated with quinolone (n=5) or oxacillin (n=2) and the mean duration was 45 days. The antimicrobial therapy was associated with pacemaker removal (n=18) or cardiac surgery (n=5). Five patients died during the early evolution of IE. Initial cure was obtained in 20 cases. IE

relapsed in one case, but cure was obtained after valvular replacement. A long, term (mean=19.5 months) follow-up was available for 12 patients. No relapse was than observed. In conclusion, fusidic acid would appear as a possible alternative for current antistaphylococcal agents used in IE.

5. Ongoing Trials

s. Urinary Tract Infections

Efficacy of Patient Self-Diagnosis and Self-Treatment for Management of Uncomplicated Recurrent Urinary Tract Infections in Women

Title	Efficacy of patient self-diagnosis and self-treatment for management of uncomplicated recurrent urinary tract infections in women.
Authors	Gupta K, Hooton TM, Stapleton A, et al.
Reference	36th Annual IDSA Meeting, Denver, CO 1998.
Background	Recurrent Urinary Tract Infection (RUT) is a common outpatient problem resulting in frequent office visits and requiring prophylactic antimicrobial use. Particularly in managed care organizations utilizing practice guidelines, patient self-diagnosis and self-treatment of RUT is increasingly being proposed as a strategy that may decrease antimicrobial use, improve patient convenience, and reduce costs. Establishing the accuracy and efficacy of this management strategy is essential for ensuring quality of care and cost-effectiveness.
Methods	We prospectively followed 122 college-age women with a history of RUT, and evaluated their accuracy in self-diagnosis, and the efficacy of self-treatment of presumed UTIs occurring over a 6–12 month period. Women with UTI symptoms collected a clean-catch urine sample and then self-initiated ofloxacin (200 mg b.i.d. x 3 d) which had been provided at study entry. Urinalysis and urine culture were performed pretherapy, and on days 10 and 30 of post-therapy.

Efficacy of Patient Self-Diagnosis and Self-Treatment
for Management of Uncomplicated Recurrent
Urinary Tract Infections in Women

(continued)

Results	60 women self-diagnosed 117 UTIs, with a mean of two episodes per women. Of these, UTI was culture confirmed in 98 (84%) episodes, sterile pyuria was present in 13 (11%) episodes, and no pyuria or bacteriuria was present in six (5%) episodes. Chlamydia ligase chain reaction was positive in one woman with sterile pyuria; none of the remaining 18 culture-negative episodes had alternative diagnoses or required further therapy. Microbiologcal and clinical failures occurred in four (3%) and one (1%) episodes respectively. Adverse events included pyelon-phritis (one), minor drug side effects (fifteen), and headache (one) and palpations (one) which required stopping the study drug.
Conclusions	Women can accurately self-diagnose and self-treat episodes of RUT, obviating the need for repeated office visits and antimicrobial prophylaxis; the strategy appears safe and effective.

5. Ongoing Trials

t. Varicella

Post-Licensure Study of Varicella Vaccine Effectiveness in a Day Care Setting

Title	Post-licensure study of varicella vaccine effectiveness in a day care setting.
Authors	Clements DA, Moreira SP, Coplan P, et al
Reference	36th Annual IDSA Meeting, Denver, CO 1998.
Summary	To document the effect of varicella vaccination, 11 day care centers in North Carolina have participated in an ongoing observational epidemiologic study. Approximately 1400 children were participating at any one point in time. Approximately 25% of the population had already had varicella, and were not eligible for consideration. During the study period from February 1, 1996 to September 1, 1997, a total of 14,392 person-months were observed. 31% (4658 person-months) of the total person-time was vaccinated. During the 19-month study period, 11 cases of varicella occurred in vaccinated children. The overall varicella incidence rate in the vaccinated group was significantly lower than that in the unvaccinated group (relative risk [RR]=0.18%; 95% confidence interval [CI] (0.1–0.33); p=0). This converts to a vaccine effectiveness of 82% (95% CI=68.5–90.8) against all forms of disease. It was 100% effective in preventing moderate to severe disease.

NOTES

NOTES

(continued)

NOTES

(continued)

NOTES

(continued)